THE ULTIMATE ANTI-INFLAMMATORY COOKBOOK

Unlock the Secret to Lasting Health with Simple, Delicious Recipes That Fight Inflammation and Boost Your Immune System Every Day

Saige Treadway

TABLE OF CONTENTS

CHAPTER 1: UNDERSTANDING THE ANTI-INFLAMMATORY DIET

Embarking on a journey toward a healthier, more vibrant self is a path filled with discovery and, often, a need for guidance. In this inaugural chapter of "The Ultimate Anti-Inflammatory Cookbook," we delve into the cornerstone of lasting health and vitality: the anti-inflammatory diet. This diet is not just about what we eat; it's about nurturing our bodies with foods that heal, protect, and revitalize. Inflammation, a natural process designed to protect our bodies, can become our adversary when it lingers longer than necessary. Chronic inflammation is quietly linked to a host of health issues, from heart disease to arthritis, and even to depression and Alzheimer's.

Our journey begins with understanding the science of inflammation and its profound impact on our well-being. Knowledge is power, and with this power, we'll explore how to harmonize our meals with our body's needs. We'll learn about the foods that are our allies in this quest, brimming with nutrients that quell inflammation, and those that are foes, exacerbating our body's stress response.

Equally important is how we stock our pantries, transforming them into treasure troves of anti-inflammatory ingredients. This chapter sets the stage for making healthful eating a seamless part of your daily routine.

As we navigate through these pages together, we're not just following recipes; we're embarking on a transformative journey. It's about embracing food as medicine—a delicious, joyful medicine that doesn't just stave off disease but enriches our lives with flavors, colors, and textures that celebrate eating as an act of self-care.

Welcome to the beginning of a journey that promises not just better health, but a more joyful, vibrant life.

1.1 THE SCIENCE OF INFLAMMATION AND YOUR HEALTH

In the heart of every health journey, there lies a fundamental truth: our bodies are complex systems, capable of healing themselves under the right conditions. At the center of this incredible system is inflammation, a response that is as essential as it is misunderstood. Often cast as the villain in our body's narrative, inflammation is actually a hero in its own right, stepping in to protect and heal. However, like any good story, there's a twist: when inflammation overstays its welcome, it can shift from protector to perpetrator, contributing to a plethora of chronic conditions that can dampen our quality of life.

Understanding inflammation requires us to delve into the body's innate intelligence. When confronted with injury or infection, our immune system springs into action, sending out inflammatory cells to the scene.

These cells act like first responders, working to eliminate the threat and initiate the healing process. This acute inflammatory response is characterized by redness, warmth, swelling, and sometimes pain—a clear signal that the body is fighting to restore balance.

But what happens when the inflammation doesn't recede? When the immune system's response becomes a constant hum rather than a temporary alarm? This is chronic inflammation, a silent turmoil simmering beneath the surface, often without the overt symptoms that accompany its acute counterpart. Chronic inflammation is the root of many modern maladies, including heart disease, diabetes, cancer, and autoimmune disorders. It's a condition fueled by a variety of factors, including stress, lack of exercise, environmental toxins, and, significantly, diet.

The foods we consume play a starring role in the story of inflammation. Just as certain substances can provoke an inflammatory response, others have the power to calm and heal. The standard American diet, rich in processed foods, sugars, and unhealthy fats, is like kindling for the fires of inflammation. Conversely, a diet abundant in fruits, vegetables, whole grains, lean proteins, and healthy fats acts as a soothing balm, quelling the flames and supporting the body's healing processes.

Herein lies the power of the anti-inflammatory diet—a way of eating that emphasizes foods known to reduce inflammation and decrease the risk of chronic disease. This approach to nutrition is not about deprivation; rather, it's a celebration of abundance. It's about filling your plate with the vibrant colors of fruits and vegetables, the heartiness of whole grains, and the essential fats found in nuts, seeds, and fish. It's a diet that delights in variety, flavor, and nourishment, grounded in the understanding that food is the most potent medicine we have.

Embarking on an anti-inflammatory diet begins with simple shifts: opting for olive oil over butter, choosing berries and leafy greens for snacks instead of chips, and favoring fish and plant-based proteins over processed meats. It's about listening to your body, noticing how different foods make you feel, and gradually steering your diet in a direction that supports your health and well-being.

The science of inflammation and its impact on health is a dynamic and evolving field. Recent studies have highlighted the interconnectedness of the gut microbiome, diet, and inflammation, offering new insights into how our dietary choices influence our overall health. A balanced gut, rich in beneficial bacteria, has been shown to play a critical role in modulating inflammation and supporting immune function. Thus, incorporating fermented foods like yogurt, kefir, and sauerkraut into your diet, along with fiber-rich foods that nourish those good bacteria, becomes an essential strategy in the fight against inflammation.

As we explore the science of inflammation and its implications for our health, it's clear that the path to wellness is paved with knowledge and nourishment.

By understanding how our diet influences inflammation, we can make informed choices that support our body's natural defenses, reduce our risk of disease, and enhance our overall vitality. In closing, the journey through the landscape of inflammation is both a personal and a universal one. Each of us has the power to influence our health trajectory through the choices we make every day, starting with what we put on our plates. The anti-inflammatory diet is more than a set of guidelines—it's a way of life that embraces food as a source of healing, joy, and connection. As we move forward in this cookbook, we'll uncover the recipes and strategies that can help you integrate this powerful approach into your life, making every meal a step toward a healthier, more vibrant you.

This exploration of the science behind inflammation and its impact on our health is just the beginning. As we venture further into the pages of this cookbook, we'll discover not only the foods that can help us combat inflammation but also how to create delicious, nourishing meals that bring joy and wellness into our daily lives. Together, we'll embark on a journey of discovery, healing, and, most importantly, delicious eating.

1.2 FOODS TO EMBRACE AND AVOID

Navigating the world of nutrition can sometimes feel like traversing a vast and complicated landscape, with every turn offering new advice on what to eat and what to avoid. In the context of an anti-inflammatory diet, this journey becomes particularly poignant, as the choices we make can directly influence our body's inflammatory response. This section aims to serve as your compass, guiding you through the foods that nourish and protect, as well as those that may provoke inflammation, steering you toward a path of wellness and vitality.

Embrace: The Anti-Inflammatory Heroes

Fruits and Vegetables: The cornerstone of any anti-inflammatory diet, fruits, and vegetables are rich in antioxidants, vitamins, minerals, and fiber, which help neutralize free radicals and reduce inflammation. Berries, leafy greens, and deeply colored vegetables like beets and sweet potatoes are particularly potent.

Whole Grains: Far from the processed flours found in white bread and pastries, whole grains provide essential nutrients and fiber that support a healthy gut and reduce inflammation. Options like quinoa, brown rice, and oats are not only versatile but also help in maintaining steady blood sugar levels.

Healthy Fats: The type of fat in your diet makes a difference. Monounsaturated and omega-3 fatty acids, found in olive oil, avocados, nuts, and fatty fish like salmon and sardines, offer anti-inflammatory benefits and support heart health.

Plant-Based Proteins: Beans, lentils, and other legumes are excellent sources of protein, fiber, and nutrients and have a lower inflammatory impact compared to some animal proteins. Incorporating these into your diet can contribute to reduced inflammation and improved gut health.

Herbs and Spices: Nature's pharmacy, herbs, and spices like turmeric, ginger, garlic, and cinnamon, are not only flavor powerhouses but also have potent anti-inflammatory properties.

Fermented Foods: Yogurt, kefir, sauerkraut, and kimchi introduce beneficial probiotics to your gut, supporting a healthy microbiome and inflammation control.

Avoid: The Inflammatory Offenders

Processed and Refined Foods: Highly processed foods, including fast food, snacks, and anything made with refined flours or sugars, can spike blood sugar levels and lead to increased inflammation.

Trans Fats and Saturated Fats: Found in fried foods, processed snacks, and some meats, these fats can trigger inflammatory responses in the body, contributing to heart disease and other health issues.

Sugar and High-Fructose Corn Syrup: Excessive sugar consumption is linked to numerous health problems, including inflammation. It's crucial to limit foods and beverages high in sugar and high-fructose corn syrup.

Red Meat and Processed Meats: While lean meats can be part of a healthy diet, consuming high amounts of red and processed meats can increase inflammation. Moderation is key, along with exploring plant-based protein sources.

Alcohol: While moderate alcohol consumption might have some health benefits, excessive intake can be detrimental, promoting inflammation and impacting liver health.

Artificial Additives: Some chemicals used to color, preserve, and flavor foods can contribute to inflammation. It's best to stick with whole, minimally processed foods to avoid these potential triggers.

In the symphony of food and health, each choice we make plays a critical note in the harmony of our body's functioning. Embracing foods that combat inflammation and avoiding those that may fuel the fire is akin to tuning our instruments, ensuring the music of our cells plays beautifully and healthfully.

Embarking on an anti-inflammatory diet isn't about strict restrictions or categorizing foods as simply good or bad; it's about balance, listening to your body, and making informed choices that support your health and well-being. It's about replacing the processed with the whole, the sugary with the naturally sweet, and the artificially flavored with the authentically delicious.

One of the most empowering aspects of this journey is the discovery of how many wonderful and flavorful options are at your fingertips. Experimenting with new fruits and vegetables, exploring the wide world of whole grains, and indulging in the rich textures and flavors of healthy fats can open up a whole new culinary landscape. It's an adventure that not only nourishes your body but also delights your palate.

As we move forward in this cookbook, you'll find recipes designed to embrace these anti-inflammatory heroes, turning them into dishes that are as satisfying as they are healthful. You'll learn how to weave these foods into your meals seamlessly, making it easier than ever to eat well and reduce inflammation. Each recipe is a step toward a healthier you, crafted with love, care, and the understanding that the best medicine is often found not in a pill bottle but at the end of your fork.

Remember, the path to reducing inflammation and enhancing your health is a journey, not a race. It's about making incremental changes that add up over time, listening to your body, and finding joy in the foods that nourish and protect you. With each bite of an anti-inflammatory meal, you're not just eating; you're taking a stand for your health, choosing to live a life filled with vitality and wellness.

1.3 BUILDING YOUR ANTI-INFLAMMATORY PANTRY

The foundation of a nourishing, anti-inflammatory lifestyle begins right in your own kitchen—more specifically, in your pantry. Consider your pantry the treasure chest of your culinary world, a place where you can reach in and pull out ingredients that not only add flavor and zest to your meals but also serve as your allies in the fight against inflammation. Building an anti-inflammatory pantry is like setting the stage for a healthier life, ensuring you have the tools and resources at your fingertips to create meals that heal, energize, and delight.

The Essentials of an Anti-Inflammatory Pantry

Whole Grains: The fiber and nutrients in whole grains play a significant role in managing inflammation. Stock your pantry with quinoa, brown rice, farro, and oats. These grains serve as versatile bases for a multitude of dishes, from morning porridges to hearty salads.

Legumes: Beans and lentils are not only high in fiber and protein but also in antioxidants. Keep a variety of dried or canned black beans, chickpeas, lentils, and kidney beans. They're perfect for soups, stews, salads, and as plant-based protein sources in your meals.

Nuts and Seeds: Almonds, walnuts, chia seeds, flaxseeds, and hemp seeds are rich in omega-3 fatty acids, which are known for their anti-inflammatory properties. They're great for snacking, adding crunch to salads, or blending into smoothies.

Healthy Fats: Olive oil is a cornerstone of the anti-inflammatory diet, thanks to its high content of monounsaturated fats and polyphenols. Avocado oil and coconut oil are also great choices for cooking and baking. Don't forget to include avocados and olives themselves for their healthy fats and phytonutrients.

Spices and Herbs: Turmeric, ginger, garlic, cinnamon, and black pepper not only add incredible flavor but also possess potent anti-inflammatory benefits. Fresh herbs like basil, parsley, and cilantro can brighten any dish and offer additional health benefits.

Vinegars and Citrus: Apple cider vinegar, balsamic vinegar, and fresh lemons and limes can add a zing to dressings, marinades, and dishes while promoting a balanced pH in the body.

Fermented Foods: Items like sauerkraut, kimchi, and miso introduce beneficial probiotics into your diet, supporting gut health and inflammation control.

Antioxidant-rich Foods: Stock up on dried or canned antioxidant-rich fruits like berries, cherries, and tomatoes. These can be fantastic additions to meals, offering a burst of flavor and a punch of anti-inflammatory power.

Sweeteners: Opt for natural sweeteners like honey and maple syrup in moderation. These can sweeten your dishes without the inflammatory effects of refined sugars.

Building Your Pantry: Practical Tips

Start Slow: Transitioning to an anti-inflammatory pantry doesn't have to happen overnight. Begin by introducing a few items at a time, gradually incorporating more as you discover what you enjoy and use most frequently.

Read Labels: When shopping, become a label detective. Opt for items with minimal ingredients, all of which you can pronounce and recognize. Avoid products with added sugars, trans fats, and artificial additives.

Bulk Buying: For non-perishable items like whole grains, legumes, nuts, and seeds, consider buying in bulk. This can be more economical and ensures you always have these staples on hand.

Organization is Key: Keep your pantry organized so that you can easily see and access all your ingredients. Use clear containers for grains, nuts, and seeds, and label them if necessary. An organized pantry invites creativity and reduces the stress of meal preparation.

Experiment with New Flavors: Use the building of your anti-inflammatory pantry as an opportunity to experiment with new ingredients and flavors. Never tried quinoa or farro? Now's the time. Curious about miso or kimchi? Add them to your pantry and explore recipes that incorporate these flavors.

Creating and maintaining an anti-inflammatory pantry is an ongoing journey, one that evolves with your tastes, preferences, and nutritional needs. As you grow more comfortable and familiar with these ingredients, you'll find that preparing healthy, anti-inflammatory meals becomes second nature. The joy of cooking comes alive when you have a pantry filled with nourishing ingredients, ready to be transformed into meals that heal the body and delight the senses.

Remember, the goal of an anti-inflammatory diet is not just about reducing inflammation; it's about enhancing your overall well-being and enjoyment of life. With each meal you prepare from your anti-inflammatory pantry, you're taking a step toward a healthier, more vibrant you. So, embrace the process of building your pantry as part of the larger journey towards health and wellness. Let your kitchen become a place of exploration, discovery, and nourishment, where every ingredient you choose brings you closer to your goals of health and vitality.

CHAPTER 2: EMBRACING THE ANTI-INFLAMMATORY LIFESTYLE

Transitioning to an anti-inflammatory lifestyle is like opening a new chapter in the book of your life, one where each page turn reveals a more vibrant, healthier you. It's about more than just modifying your diet; it's a holistic approach that weaves the threads of nutritious eating, mindful living, and joyful movement into the fabric of your daily life.

In this chapter, we delve into the heart of embracing the anti-inflammatory lifestyle, providing you with the tools and inspiration needed to make this transition not only achievable but also deeply rewarding. It's about understanding that change doesn't happen overnight and that every small step you take is a leap towards a more energetic, pain-free existence.

Here, we explore strategies for integrating anti-inflammatory foods into your meals in a way that feels natural and enjoyable. We'll talk about how to shop smartly, choosing ingredients that nourish and satisfy, and how to set up your kitchen for success, turning it into a haven for healthful cooking. But it's not just about what you eat; it's also about cultivating a mindset that supports your journey. Mindful eating, stress management, and connecting with your body's needs become key components of your daily routine.

This chapter aims to guide you through creating a lifestyle that supports your well-being from the inside out, making every choice an affirmation of your commitment to living well. Join us on this journey, and discover the joy and abundance that comes from embracing the anti-inflammatory lifestyle.

2.1 MAKING THE SHIFT

Transitioning to an anti-inflammatory lifestyle is akin to embarking on a thrilling journey toward a vibrant and healthier self. It's a path that introduces you to a world of new tastes, textures, and colors, bringing a sense of renewal to your meals and, by extension, to your life. The process is gradual, filled with small, manageable steps that collectively lead to a profound transformation in how you feel, eat, and think about food.

Embracing this change is the first and most crucial step. It's about viewing this lifestyle shift not as a restriction but as an exciting opportunity to explore and enjoy a bounty of wholesome, inflammation-fighting foods. Slowly integrating these foods into your diet helps make the transition smoother and more enjoyable. You don't need to empty your pantry and start from scratch overnight. Instead, focus on adding vibrant fruits, vegetables, whole grains, and lean proteins to your meals bit by bit.

Gaining a solid understanding of why certain foods are preferred in an anti-inflammatory diet empowers you to make informed choices.

Recognizing the role of chronic inflammation in health issues and how specific dietary choices can mitigate this risk is key. Opting for nutrient-rich foods like leafy greens and fatty fish becomes a meaningful, intentional act of self-care.

Creativity in the kitchen through the art of substitution can transform your meal prep into an adventure. Cravings for traditional favorites can be met with healthier alternatives that don't skimp on flavor. Think avocado for butter in baking or zucchini noodles in place of pasta. These swaps not only introduce you to new flavors but also keep your diet varied and exciting.

Mindfulness extends beyond meditation to how and what you eat. Adopting a mindful approach to eating—savoring each bite, listening to your body's cues, and enjoying the moment—can significantly enhance your relationship with food. This practice helps in appreciating the natural flavors of anti-inflammatory foods and in making mealtime a nourishing experience for both body and soul.

Planning your meals is an invaluable strategy that anchors this new lifestyle. It ensures that you have a roadmap for the week, making it less likely you'll reach for convenience foods. Starting with planning a few days ahead and gradually increasing to a full week can make a world of difference. Preparing ingredients in advance further simplifies the process, making healthy eating a practical part of your busy schedule.

Change is a journey, not a sprint. Emphasizing gradual, sustainable changes rather than drastic overhauls helps integrate the anti-inflammatory diet into your life without feeling overwhelmed. Small victories, like opting for healthier snacks or adding an extra serving of vegetables to your plate, pave the way for more significant, lasting changes.

Building a support network can provide encouragement, accountability, and shared experiences. Whether it's through family, friends, or online communities, connecting with others on a similar path can offer invaluable support and motivation. Sharing your goals and progress can make the journey more enjoyable and less daunting.

Listening to your body is essential as you adapt to this new way of eating. Everyone's body reacts differently to dietary changes, and what works for one person may not work for another. Paying attention to how you feel after eating certain foods allows you to tailor your diet to your body's unique needs.

Flexibility is crucial in maintaining an anti-inflammatory lifestyle, especially during social events or while traveling. Rather than seeing these situations as setbacks, view them as opportunities to make the best possible choices within the given context. The aim is consistency over perfection, focusing on the overall dietary pattern rather than isolated incidents.

In essence, making the shift to an anti-inflammatory lifestyle is a journey filled with learning, growth, and discovery.

It's about more than just the food on your plate; it's a comprehensive approach to well-being that embraces nutritious eating, mindful living, and the joy of discovering new ways to nourish your body. Each step forward is a step towards a healthier, more vibrant you, making every meal an opportunity to nurture not just your body, but your overall quality of life. Welcome to this transformative path, where each choice reflects a commitment to your health and well-being.

2.2 MINDFUL EATING

In the journey toward embracing an anti-inflammatory lifestyle, mindful eating emerges as a beacon, guiding us to not only what we eat but how we eat. It's about cultivating a relationship with food that transcends the mere act of eating to fill hunger—it's about experiencing food with all our senses, understanding its journey from earth to plate, and appreciating its nourishment of our bodies and souls. This connection deepens our appreciation for the abundance nature offers, fostering gratitude and a profound sense of well-being.

Mindful eating is an invitation to slow down and savor life. In our fast-paced world, meals often become another task to check off the list. We eat distractedly, disconnected from the experience, which can lead to overeating and a disconnection from our body's natural cues. By engaging fully with our meals, we learn to listen to our hunger signals, recognize when we're satisfied, and discover the true pleasure of eating.

At the heart of mindful eating is the practice of presence. This means sitting down for meals without the distraction of screens or work, focusing entirely on the experience of eating. Notice the colors, textures, and aromas of your food; chew slowly and savor each bite. This practice not only enhances the enjoyment of your meal but also aids digestion and satisfaction, allowing the body to signal fullness effectively.

Mindful eating also involves an awareness of our food's origins. It encourages us to consider where our food comes from, the journey it has taken to reach our plates, and the effort of those who grew, harvested, and prepared it. This awareness builds a deeper respect for our nourishment, prompting choices that are more in alignment with an anti-inflammatory lifestyle—choices that favor fresh, whole foods over processed alternatives.

The practice of mindful eating also opens up a space for emotional awareness and healing. Many of us have complex relationships with food, often using it to comfort, reward, or punish ourselves.

Mindful eating allows us to explore these patterns without judgment, understanding the emotional triggers that lead to mindless eating. By acknowledging these habits, we can begin to heal our relationship with food, choosing to eat for nourishment rather than as an emotional response.

Mindful eating doesn't mean you must eat perfectly at every meal. Rather, it's about bringing consciousness to your eating habits, making intentional choices that align with your health goals, and forgiving yourself when you stray from these intentions. It's a practice of returning, again and again, to the present moment and choosing what serves your body and mind best.

Incorporating mindful eating into your life doesn't require drastic changes; it begins with small, manageable steps. Start by dedicating one meal a day to eat mindfully, free from distractions. Gradually, as this practice becomes ingrained, expand it to more meals and snacks. Over time, you'll find that these moments of mindfulness spill over into other areas of your life, enhancing your overall well-being.

The journey towards mindful eating is also a journey of discovery—discovering new flavors, textures, and combinations that delight the senses. It encourages experimentation and creativity in the kitchen, leading to a richer, more diverse diet that supports your anti-inflammatory lifestyle. It turns mealtime into an exploration, where each dish offers an opportunity to connect with your body and the world around you.

Mindful eating also fosters a sense of community. Sharing meals with others becomes a shared experience of mindfulness, where the act of eating together deepens relationships and creates a space for connection. It's an invitation to come together in appreciation, not just of the food but of the company and the moment.

Ultimately, mindful eating is a form of self-care. It's an acknowledgment of the importance of nourishing not just the body but also the mind and spirit. It's a commitment to living fully, with awareness and appreciation for the present moment and the nourishment it offers. As you embrace mindful eating, you'll discover not just a path to a healthier you, but a path to a more connected, joyful, and mindful life.

As we continue our exploration of the anti-inflammatory lifestyle, let mindful eating be your guide. Let it transform not just the way you eat, but the way you live, leading you towards greater health, happiness, and harmony. Remember, this journey is not just about the destination but about savoring each step along the way.

2.3 Anti-Inflammatory Lifestyle Beyond the Diet

Embracing an anti-inflammatory lifestyle extends far beyond the realm of diet, weaving into the fabric of our daily lives through practices that nurture both the mind and body. This holistic approach is a multifaceted journey, touching upon stress management, physical activity, sleep quality, and the richness of human connection, each contributing to a well-rounded and vibrant state of health.

Stress, an omnipresent force in modern life, plays a significant role in inflammation. Tackling this unseen adversary with mindfulness techniques, yoga, or simply deep-breathing exercises can recalibrate the body's response, fostering a state of calm resilience. These practices act as anchors, steadying us amidst life's tumultuous seas and mitigating the inflammatory responses triggered by chronic stress.

Physical activity, too, is a cornerstone of this lifestyle, celebrated not as a duty but as a joyous expression of living. The secret lies in discovering activities that thrill and engage you, transforming exercise from a mundane task into a source of pleasure. Regular movement, from gentle walks to the energetic pulse of dance, harnesses exercise's natural anti-inflammatory effects, enhancing both mood and physical well-being.

Sleep's role in our health is profound, with its restorative power acting as a nightly reset for the body's inflammatory processes. Cultivating practices that promote restful sleep, such as maintaining a consistent sleep schedule and crafting a tranquil bedtime environment, can significantly amplify the body's ability to combat inflammation. It's in the embrace of quality sleep that the body finds its balance, repairing and rejuvenating itself.

The fabric of our lives is also woven with the threads of connection and community. These human bonds are essential, nourishing our emotional health and acting as a buffer against stress. Engaging in meaningful relationships and community activities enriches our lives, providing a sense of belonging and support that is crucial for mental and physical health.

As we navigate this journey, integrating mindful technology use becomes increasingly important. Setting boundaries around screen time and engaging in regular digital detoxes can mitigate technology-induced stress, allowing for more genuine connections with ourselves and those around us.

Our environment, too, plays a pivotal role in our health. By choosing natural products and supporting sustainable practices, we reduce our exposure to harmful toxins and contribute to a healthier planet. These choices reflect a broader commitment to living in harmony with our environment, recognizing its impact on our well-being.

At the heart of this lifestyle is the cultivation of joy and gratitude. It's about savoring the moment, embracing the abundance around us, and practicing gratitude for the simple pleasures in life. This positive outlook is not just uplifting; it's transformative, reducing stress and promoting a deep sense of fulfillment.

Embarking on the path to an anti-inflammatory lifestyle is to embrace a journey of discovery and growth. It's a commitment to enriching not just our bodies but our entire being, making choices that reflect our deepest values and aspirations. It's about progress, not perfection, and finding joy in the journey itself.

This lifestyle is a comprehensive approach to well-being, blending the physical with the emotional and the environmental, each aspect supporting and enhancing the others. It's a way of life that invites us to live more fully, more consciously, and more joyously, with every choice and every action aligned with our health and happiness.

As we venture deeper into this lifestyle, we learn that living anti-inflammatory is not merely about avoiding certain foods but about embracing a way of life that fosters health, harmony, and happiness. It's a journey that challenges us to grow, to adapt, and to flourish, discovering along the way that the true essence of well-being lies in the balance and richness of our daily lives.

In embracing this holistic approach, we find ourselves not just following a diet but living a life infused with awareness, joy, and a deep connection to the world around us. This is the true heart of the anti-inflammatory lifestyle—a vibrant tapestry of practices that nourish the body, soothe the mind, and fill the soul with joy.

2.4 KITCHEN SETUP FOR SUCCESS

As you embark on your anti-inflammatory journey, your kitchen becomes more than just a place to cook—it transforms into a sanctuary where wellness begins. Setting it up for success is pivotal, laying the groundwork for a lifestyle that's as nourishing as it is delightful. This preparation involves more than just stocking up on ingredients; it's about creating an environment that inspires health, efficiency, and joy in every meal you prepare.

The essence of a well-prepared kitchen lies in its simplicity. Start by decluttering, removing anything that doesn't serve your new lifestyle. This act of clearing out not only makes space for the new but also simplifies your cooking processes, making healthy choices easier and more accessible. Essentials like a good set of knives, durable chopping boards, and reliable cookware become your allies, each item selected for its role in crafting nourishing meals.

Consider the storage of your tools and ingredients as part of this simplification. Transparent, airtight containers not only preserve the freshness of your ingredients but also offer visual cues to what's available, encouraging their use and minimizing waste. This visibility is crucial, guiding your daily choices towards the freshest, most nutritious options.

The heart of your anti-inflammatory kitchen is undoubtedly your pantry. Stock it with staples that support your health goals: whole grains, legumes, nuts, seeds, and a bounty of spices and herbs that bring both flavor and anti-inflammatory benefits to your dishes. Quality oils for cooking and dressing salads, like extra virgin olive oil, become indispensable, enriching your meals with healthy fats.

The Cold Keepers: Fridge and Freezer

Your refrigerator and freezer are your gateways to fresh, vibrant ingredients. Prioritize spaces for vegetables, fruits, lean proteins, and probiotic-rich foods. These components of your diet are foundational, supporting your body's natural anti-inflammatory processes. The freezer, meanwhile, offers a haven for meal prep, allowing you to store batches of wholesome meals for days when time is scarce.

Flavor's Architects: Herbs and Spices

Allocating a specific area for your herbs and spices not only keeps your kitchen organized but also invites culinary creativity. These natural enhancers reduce the need for salt or sugar, offering a way to elevate the nutritional and taste profile of your meals effortlessly. Experimenting with different combinations can transform simple ingredients into exquisite dishes that delight the senses.

A kitchen that supports an anti-inflammatory lifestyle is one where everything has its place, designed for efficiency and ease. Implement systems that let you access what you need without hassle, reducing the friction between you and your next healthful meal. Labels, transparent storage, and a logical arrangement of items streamline your cooking process, making the preparation of nutritious meals an integral part of your routine.

Modern kitchen gadgets offer more than convenience; they provide new ways to prepare your meals while preserving or even enhancing their nutritional value. Tools like slow cookers, pressure cookers, and blenders support your anti-inflammatory diet, making it easier to incorporate whole, unprocessed foods into your daily meals.

Creating a kitchen you love is about more than functionality—it's about inspiration. Personalize your space with elements that make you feel happy and motivated, whether that's through decor, music, or anything else that enhances your cooking experience. This personal touch transforms your kitchen from a mere room into a source of joy and creativity.

Your kitchen, much like your journey, is ever evolving. Stay open to making adjustments to your setup and tools as you discover what works best for you. This flexibility ensures your kitchen remains a true reflection of your commitment to an anti-inflammatory lifestyle, adapting as you grow and learn.

In crafting a kitchen setup for success, you're doing more than organizing a space—you're building a foundation for a lifestyle that cherishes health and well-being. It's here, in the heart of your home, that you'll craft meals that nourish, heal, and bring joy. Each ingredient, each tool, and each meal becomes a step on your path to wellness, a testament to the transformative power of an anti-inflammatory lifestyle. Through this careful preparation, your kitchen becomes not just a place to cook, but a sanctuary for health, creativity, and joy, embodying the essence of your journey toward a vibrant, flourishing life.

2.5 ENGAGING FAMILY AND FRIENDS

Embracing an anti-inflammatory lifestyle transforms your journey into a communal voyage, enriched by the participation of family and friends. This collective endeavor not only deepens personal commitments but also spreads the seeds of wellness within your closest circles, creating a shared tapestry of health and vitality. Here, we explore ways to bring those closest to you along on this enriching path, turning individual pursuits into shared adventures that strengthen bonds and foster communal well-being.

Cooking becomes a collaborative art when you invite loved ones into the kitchen. This shared space turns meal preparation into a collective experience that's as nourishing for the relationships as it is for the body. Together, you delve into the joy of creating dishes that are both healthful and delicious, exchanging stories and laughter, and making memories that bind you closer. This practice not only demystifies the anti-inflammatory lifestyle but also showcases the abundance and flavor that define it, proving that choosing health does not mean sacrificing taste or enjoyment.

Education plays a pivotal role in this shared journey. By disseminating knowledge about the benefits and principles of anti-inflammatory eating among your circle, you ignite curiosity and inspire informed choices.

Casual discussions, shared articles, and resources illuminate the science behind the diet, encouraging everyone to explore and adopt practices that resonate with their individual health goals. This ongoing dialogue fosters an environment of mutual learning and support, where everyone is empowered to make choices that align with their well-being.

Hosting gatherings centered around anti-inflammatory cuisine offers a unique opportunity to dispel myths and demonstrate the diet's diversity and deliciousness. Menus crafted with care show that food can be both healing and indulgent, broadening perspectives and enticing even the most skeptical guests. These events become platforms for conversation and conversion, gently introducing the principles of anti-inflammatory eating in a setting that is social, relaxed, and inclusive.

Recognizing the personal nature of each individual's health journey is crucial. Approach conversations with empathy, understanding that everyone's path to wellness is unique. Small steps toward a healthier lifestyle are celebrated, acknowledging the effort and intention behind each choice. This gentle encouragement fosters a positive environment where change is inspired, not imposed, allowing each person to navigate their own journey at their own pace.

Cultivating a support network enriches the anti-inflammatory lifestyle, providing a sense of community and shared purpose. Whether through formal meetings or casual get-togethers, these connections offer encouragement, exchange of ideas, and mutual support. They remind us that we are not alone in our quest for health, providing a foundation of companionship and motivation that bolsters resilience and commitment.

The journey will undoubtedly present challenges, from navigating temptations to finding anti-inflammatory options in social settings. Sharing these experiences with your circle invites collective problem-solving and support, turning obstacles into opportunities for growth and strengthening. This communal resilience transforms challenges into shared victories, deepening connections and reinforcing the collective commitment to wellness.

Celebrating successes with your loved ones amplifies the joy of the journey. Whether it's the discovery of a new favorite recipe, an improvement in health markers, or the successful incorporation of a challenging ingredient, these moments of triumph are magnified when shared. They not only reinforce the benefits of the anti-inflammatory lifestyle but also inspire others to pursue their wellness goals.

Introducing flexibility and fun into the diet encourages exploration and creativity, making the lifestyle enjoyable and sustainable. Themed cooking nights, recipe exchanges, and culinary challenges infuse the journey with excitement, inviting everyone to engage with anti-inflammatory eating in a way that feels playful and exploratory.

Leading by example is perhaps the most powerful method of engagement. Living your commitment to an anti-inflammatory lifestyle with enthusiasm and integrity serves as a beacon for others, demonstrating the tangible benefits of such a lifestyle. Your vitality and wellness become a testament to the lifestyle's efficacy, inspiring those around you through the compelling evidence of your own transformation.

At its core, involving family and friends in your anti-inflammatory lifestyle is an act of communal nurturing. It's about extending the care you have for yourself to those you love, sharing knowledge, support, and the joy of healthful living. This journey, embarked upon together, not only enhances your own path to wellness but also weaves a collective narrative of health, connection, and shared joy. Through cooking, learning, celebrating, and supporting each other, you create a vibrant community culture centered on well-being, enriching the lives of all involved and making the journey an inclusive celebration of health.

CHAPTER 3: BREAKFAST RECIPES

Rise and shine to a new dawn of vitality and wellness! Chapter 2 opens the door to a world where breakfast isn't just the first meal of the day—it's a foundational step in nurturing your body and combating inflammation from the moment you wake. Here, we've carefully curated a collection of breakfast recipes that are not only a delight to your taste buds but also a boon to your health.

Each recipe is crafted with the understanding that mornings can be hectic. We aim to simplify your routine without compromising on nutrition or taste. From energizing smoothies that you can whip up in minutes to savory skillets filled with anti-inflammatory goodness, these breakfasts are designed to fit into your busy life while setting a positive tone for the day ahead.

Imagine starting your day with foods that not only satisfy your hunger but also soothe your body, reducing inflammation and boosting your immune system. Whether you're sitting down to a leisurely breakfast with family or grabbing a quick bite before you dash out the door, these meals will ensure you're well-nourished and ready to face the day.

Breakfast is often called the most important meal of the day, and in the context of an anti-inflammatory diet, this couldn't be truer. The recipes in this chapter are your first step each day towards a healthier, happier you. They say that how you start your morning can set the tone for the entire day—let's make it a harmonious one, filled with health, energy, and joy.

3.1 ENERGIZING SMOOTHIES AND JUICES

GOLDEN TURMERIC MORNING KICK

P.T.: 5 min | **C.T.:** 0 min

M. of C.: Blending | **Serves:** 2

Ingr.: 1 C. unsweetened almond milk

- ½ C. orange juice, freshly squeezed

- 1 banana, ripe

- ½ tsp ground turmeric

- ¼ tsp ground cinnamon

- 1 Tbls chia seeds

- 1 tsp honey, raw

- A pinch of black pepper

Proc.: Combine all ingredients in a blender

- Blend on high until smooth and creamy

- Serve immediately

N.V.: Calories: 145, Fat: 2g, Carbs: 30g, Protein: 3g, Sugar: 17g

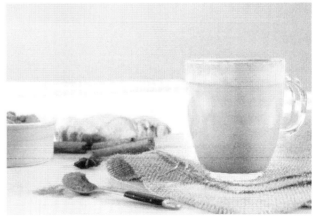

BERRY ANTI-INFLAMMATORY BLAST

P.T.: 7 min | **C.T.:** 0 min

M. of C.: Blending | **Serves:** 2

Ingr.: 1 C. mixed berries, frozen (blueberries, strawberries, raspberries)

- 1 C. spinach, fresh

- 1 C. coconut water

- ½ avocado

- 1 Tbls flaxseeds

- 2 tsp lemon juice, freshly squeezed

- 1 Tbls almond butter

Proc.: Place all ingredients in a blender

- Blend until smooth

- Taste and adjust sweetness, if necessary, with a bit more lemon juice

N.V.: Calories: 220, Fat: 11g, Carbs: 28g, Protein: 5g, Sugar: 15g

GREEN GINGER-PEACH ENERGY

P.T.: 6 min | **C.T.:** 0 min

M. of C.: Blending | **Serves:** 2

Ingr.: 2 C. spinach, fresh

- 1 C. peaches, sliced and frozen

- 1 banana, ripe

- ½ inch ginger, fresh, peeled and minced

- 1 C. almond milk

- 1 tsp flaxseed oil

- 1 Tbls honey, raw

Proc.: Add spinach, peaches, banana, and ginger to the blender

- Pour in almond milk and add flaxseed oil and honey

- Blend on high until smooth

- Serve chilled

N.V.: Calories: 190, Fat: 4g, Carbs: 38g, Protein: 3g, Sugar: 25g

ANTIOXIDANT ACAI REFRESHER

P.T.: 8 min | **C.T.:** 0 min

M. of C.: Blending | **Serves:** 2

Ingr.: 1 packet acai berry puree, unsweetened

- 1 C. mixed berries, fresh

- 1 C. unsweetened coconut milk

- 1 Tbls pumpkin seeds

- ½ banana

- 1 tsp matcha powder

- 1 Tbls chia seeds

- 1 Tbls maple syrup, pure

Proc.: Thaw acai puree slightly

- Combine acai puree with the berries, coconut milk, and banana in a blender

- Add pumpkin seeds, matcha powder, chia seeds, and maple syrup

- Blend until smooth

- Serve chilled or over ice

N.V.: Calories: 180, Fat: 7g, Carbs: 26g, Protein: 4g, Sugar: 14g

SPIRULINA SUNRISE SMOOTHIE

P.T.: 5 min | **C.T.:** 0 min

M. of C.: Blending | **Serves:** 2

Ingr.: 1 C. coconut water

- 1 banana, ripe

- 1/2 C. pineapple chunks, fresh or frozen

- 1/2 C. mango chunks, fresh or frozen

- 1 tsp spirulina powder

- 1 Tbls chia seeds

- 1 Tbls honey, optional

- Ice cubes, as needed

Proc.: Place all ingredients in a blender

- Blend on high until smooth and creamy

- Taste and adjust sweetness with honey if desired

- Add ice cubes for a colder smoothie and blend again until desired consistency is reached

- Serve immediately in chilled glasses

N.V.: Calories: 180, Fat: 1g, Carbs: 42g, Protein: 3g, Sugar: 29g

3.2 WHOLESOME PORRIDGES AND OATMEALS

CINNAMON SPICED QUINOA PORRIDGE

P.T.: 10 min | **C.T.:** 15 min

M. of C.: Simmering | **Serves:** 2

Ingr.: 1 C. quinoa, rinsed

- 2 C. almond milk

- 1 cinnamon stick

- 1 apple, peeled and grated

- 2 Tbls walnuts, chopped

- 1 Tbls chia seeds

- 1 tsp vanilla extract

- 2 tsp honey, raw

- ¼ tsp ground nutmeg

Proc.: Combine quinoa, almond milk, and cinnamon stick in a saucepan

- Bring to a boil, then reduce heat and simmer, covered, for 15 min

- Remove from heat and discard cinnamon stick

- Stir in grated apple, walnuts, chia seeds, vanilla extract, honey, and nutmeg

- Serve warm

N.V.: Calories: 320, Fat: 9g, Carbs: 50g, Protein: 11g, Sugar: 10g

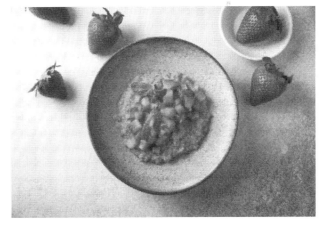

ANTI-INFLAMMATORY OATS WITH TURMERIC AND GINGER

P.T.: 5 min | **C.T.:** 10 min

M. of C.: Simmering | **Serves:** 2

Ingr.: 1 C. rolled oats

- 2 C. coconut milk
- ½ tsp ground turmeric
- ¼ tsp ground ginger
- 1 Tbls flaxseed meal
- 1 banana, sliced
- 1 Tbls almond slices
- 1 tsp honey, raw
- A pinch of black pepper

Proc.: Combine rolled oats, coconut milk, turmeric, ginger, and flaxseed meal in a saucepan

- Bring to a boil, then reduce heat and simmer for 10 min, stirring occasionally

- Serve topped with banana slices, almond slices, a drizzle of honey, and a pinch of black pepper

N.V.: Calories: 350, Fat: 14g, Carbs: 48g, Protein: 8g, Sugar: 15g

BERRY BUCKWHEAT BREAKFAST BOWL

P.T.: 10 min | **C.T.:** 20 min

M. of C.: Boiling | **Serves:** 2

Ingr.: 1 C. buckwheat groats

- 2½ C. water
- ½ C. mixed berries, fresh
- 2 Tbls hemp seeds
- 1 Tbls pumpkin seeds
- 1 Tbls sunflower seeds
- 2 tsp maple syrup, pure
- ½ tsp vanilla extract
- A pinch of salt

Proc.: Rinse buckwheat groats under cold water

- Combine groats, water, and salt in a saucepan and bring to a boil

- Reduce heat, cover, and simmer for 20 min or until groats are tender

- Remove from heat and stir in vanilla extract

- Serve topped with berries, hemp seeds, pumpkin seeds, sunflower seeds, and a drizzle of maple syrup

N.V.: Calories: 330, Fat: 9g, Carbs: 55g, Protein: 12g, Sugar: 10g

TURMERIC GINGER OATMEAL

P.T.: 10 min | **C.T.:** 15 min

M. of C.: Simmering | **Serves:** 2

Ingr.: 1 C. rolled oats

- 2 C. almond milk
- 1 tsp turmeric powder
- 1/2 tsp ginger powder
- 1/4 tsp cinnamon
- 1 Tbls flaxseed meal
- 1 Tbls honey or maple syrup
- 1 apple, diced
- 2 Tbls walnuts, chopped
- A pinch of black pepper

Proc.: Combine rolled oats and almond milk in a medium saucepan and bring to a simmer over medium heat

- Stir in turmeric, ginger, cinnamon, and flaxseed meal

- Reduce heat and simmer for 10-15 minutes, stirring occasionally, until oats are tender and the porridge has thickened

- Remove from heat and stir in honey or maple syrup

- Serve topped with diced apple and chopped walnuts, with a pinch of black pepper sprinkled on top

N.V.: Calories: 300, Fat: 9g, Carbs: 48g, Protein: 8g, Sugar: 16g

3.3 SAVORY BREAKFAST BOWLS AND SKILLETS

MEDITERRANEAN CHICKPEA SKILLET

P.T.: 10 min | **C.T.:** 20 min

M. of C.: Sautéing | **Serves:** 2

Ingr.: 1 Tbls olive oil

- 1 small onion, diced

- 2 cloves garlic, minced

- 1 red bell pepper, diced

- 1 C. chickpeas, cooked and drained

- 1 C. spinach, fresh

- 4 eggs

- 1 tsp smoked paprika

- ½ tsp cumin

- Salt and pepper to taste

- 2 Tbls parsley, chopped

- 1 avocado, sliced

Proc.: Heat olive oil in a skillet over medium heat

- Sauté onion, garlic, and bell pepper until softened

- Add chickpeas, spinach, smoked paprika, cumin, salt, and pepper, cooking until spinach is wilted

- Create four wells in the mixture and crack an egg into each

- Cover and cook until eggs are set to your liking

- Serve garnished with parsley and sliced avocado

N.V.: Calories: 400, Fat: 24g, Carbs: 34g, Protein: 20g, Sugar: 7g

SWEET POTATO AND KALE HASH

P.T.: 15 min | **C.T.:** 25 min

M. of C.: Roasting | **Serves:** 2

Ingr.: 2 sweet potatoes, cubed

- 1 Tbls coconut oil, melted

- 1 tsp turmeric

- ½ tsp garlic powder

- Salt and pepper to taste

- 2 C. kale, chopped

- 4 eggs

- 1 avocado, sliced

- 1 Tbls pumpkin seeds

Proc.: Preheat oven to 400°F (200°C)

- Toss sweet potatoes with coconut oil, turmeric, garlic powder, salt, and pepper, and spread on a baking sheet

- Roast for 20 min, then add kale, tossing to combine, and roast for another 5 min

- Fry eggs to your preference in a skillet

- Serve hash topped with fried eggs, sliced avocado, and sprinkle with pumpkin seeds

N.V.: Calories: 450, Fat: 27g, Carbs: 38g, Protein: 18g, Sugar: 5g

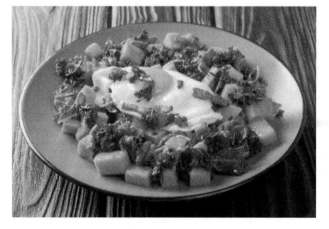

ZUCCHINI AND TOMATO FRITTATA

P.T.: 10 min | **C.T.:** 15 min

M. of C.: Baking | **Serves:** 2

Ingr.: 4 eggs

- 1 small zucchini, thinly sliced

- 1 tomato, sliced

- ½ onion, thinly sliced

- 1 Tbls olive oil

- ¼ C. almond milk

- Salt and pepper to taste

- 1 tsp Italian seasoning

- ¼ C. goat cheese, crumbled

- 2 Tbls basil, chopped

Proc.: Preheat oven to 375°F (190°C)

- Sauté onion and zucchini in olive oil over medium heat until tender

- Whisk together eggs, almond milk, salt, pepper, and Italian seasoning

- Pour egg mixture over sautéed vegetables, then lay tomato slices on top

- Sprinkle with goat cheese

- Bake in the oven for 15 min or until set

- Garnish with chopped basil before serving

N.V.: Calories: 320, Fat: 22g, Carbs: 10g, Protein: 20g, Sugar: 6g

ANTI-INFLAMMATORY AVOCADO AND EGG BREAKFAST BOWL

P.T.: 10 min | **C.T.:** 5 min

M. of C.: Cooking | **Serves:** 2

Ingr.: 1 avocado, halved and pitted

- 4 eggs

- 2 cups spinach

- 1 cup quinoa, cooked

- 1 tablespoon olive oil

- 1/2 teaspoon turmeric

- 1/4 teaspoon garlic powder

- Salt and pepper to taste

- 1/4 cup cherry tomatoes, halved

- 2 tablespoons pumpkin seeds

Proc.: Heat olive oil in a skillet over medium heat

- Add spinach and sauté until wilted

- Season with turmeric, garlic powder, salt, and pepper

- Divide cooked quinoa between two bowls

- In the same skillet, fry eggs to your preference

- Place eggs and sautéed spinach over quinoa

- Arrange avocado halves and cherry tomatoes around the bowl

- Sprinkle with pumpkin seeds before serving

N.V.: Calories: 420, Fat: 25g, Carbs: 35g, Protein: 20g, Sugar: 3g

CHAPTER 4: SALAD RECIPES

Embarking on a journey through the vibrant world of salads, we dive into the heart of what makes eating both a pleasure and a powerful tool for nurturing our well-being. In this chapter, we unveil an array of salad recipes that aren't just about tossing greens in a bowl but about creating symphonies of flavors and textures that invigorate the palate and soothe the body.

Salads, often underestimated, are a cornerstone of the anti-inflammatory diet, offering a canvas to paint with the broad spectrum of nature's colors and nutrients. From the deep greens of spinach and kale to the bright reds of tomatoes and the earthy tones of legumes, every color represents a different set of phytonutrients, working in harmony to reduce inflammation and enhance our immune response.

Here, we'll explore the art of balancing flavors and textures, combining crisp vegetables, soft grains, creamy dressings, and crunchy toppings to achieve meals that are as satisfying as they are healthful. We'll venture beyond the traditional, incorporating protein-packed ingredients and innovative dressings that turn our salads into hearty mains or refreshing sides.

Whether you're looking for a light lunch option, a robust dinner salad, or something to share at your next gathering, these recipes are designed to impress your taste buds and support your health. Each creation is a testament to the fact that nourishing your body doesn't have to be a chore—it can be an exciting, flavorful adventure.

As we journey through this chapter, remember that each recipe is a stepping stone towards a lifestyle where food is your ally in maintaining vitality and combating inflammation. Let's embrace the bounty of our gardens and markets, and transform simple ingredients into dishes that delight and heal.

4.1 LEAFY GREENS AND VIBRANT VEGGIES

KALE AND QUINOA RAINBOW SALAD

P.T.: 15 min | **C.T.:** 0 min

M. of C.: No Cooking | **Serves:** 4

Ingr.: 2 C. kale, finely chopped

- 1 C. quinoa, cooked and cooled

- 1 red bell pepper, diced

- 1 yellow bell pepper, diced

- 1 orange carrot, julienned

- ½ C. red cabbage, shredded

- ¼ C. almonds, sliced

- ¼ C. dried cranberries

- For the dressing: 3 Tbls olive oil

- 1 Tbls apple cider vinegar

- 1 tsp honey

- 1 tsp Dijon mustard

- Salt and pepper to taste

Proc.: Whisk together dressing ingredients in a small bowl

- In a large salad bowl, combine kale, quinoa, bell peppers, carrot, cabbage, almonds, and cranberries

- Pour dressing over salad and toss to coat evenly

- Serve immediately

N.V.: Calories: 280, Fat: 14g, Carbs: 34g, Protein: 8g, Sugar: 9g

BEETROOT AND SPINACH DETOX SALAD

P.T.: 20 min | **C.T.:** 0 min

M. of C.: No Cooking | **Serves:** 2

Ingr.: 2 medium beetroots, raw, peeled and grated

- 2 C. baby spinach, fresh

- 1 avocado, diced

- ½ C. walnuts, chopped

- 2 Tbls pumpkin seeds

- For the dressing: 2 Tbls flaxseed oil

- 2 tsp lemon juice

- 1 tsp maple syrup

- 1 garlic clove, minced

- Salt and pepper to taste

Proc.: Combine dressing ingredients in a jar and shake well

- In a salad bowl, mix together beetroots, spinach, avocado, walnuts, and pumpkin seeds

- Drizzle dressing over the salad and toss gently to combine

- Serve fresh

N.V.: Calories: 360, Fat: 26g, Carbs: 30g, Protein: 9g, Sugar: 12g

ASIAN STYLE SLAW WITH GINGER DRESSING

P.T.: 10 min | **C.T.:** 0 min

M. of C.: No Cooking | **Serves:** 4

Ingr.: 3 C. Napa cabbage, shredded

- 1 C. carrot, julienned

- 1 red bell pepper, thinly sliced

- 1 C. cucumber, julienned

- ½ C. cilantro, chopped

- ¼ C. green onions, sliced

- For the dressing: 3 Tbls sesame oil

- 2 Tbls rice vinegar

- 1 Tbls soy sauce

- 1 Tbls honey

- 1 Tbls ginger, grated

- 1 garlic clove, minced

- 1 tsp sesame seeds

Proc.: Whisk together dressing ingredients until well combined

- In a large bowl, combine all salad ingredients

- Pour dressing over salad and toss well to coat

- Sprinkle sesame seeds on top before serving

N.V.: Calories: 180, Fat: 14g, Carbs: 13g, Protein: 3g, Sugar: 8g

WATERMELON AND FETA SALAD WITH MINT

P.T.: 15 min | **C.T.:** 0 min

M. of C.: No Cooking | **Serves:** 4

Ingr.: 4 C. watermelon, cubed

- 1 C. feta cheese, crumbled

- ½ C. mint leaves, torn

- ¼ C. red onion, thinly sliced

- 2 Tbls olive oil

- 1 Tbls balsamic vinegar

- Salt and pepper to taste

Proc.: In a large salad bowl, combine watermelon, feta cheese, mint leaves, and red onion

- In a small bowl, whisk together olive oil, balsamic vinegar, salt, and pepper to create the dressing

- Drizzle the dressing over the salad and gently toss to combine

- Chill before serving

N.V.: Calories: 190, Fat: 12g, Carbs: 17g, Protein: 5g, Sugar: 14g

KALE AND ROASTED SWEET POTATO SALAD

P.T.: 20 min | **C.T.:** 25 min

M. of C.: Roasting | **Serves:** 4

Ingr.: 2 large sweet potatoes, cubed

- 1 Tbls olive oil

- Salt and pepper to taste

- 4 cups kale, stems removed and leaves chopped

- 1/4 cup dried cranberries

- 1/4 cup walnuts, toasted and chopped

- For the dressing: 2 Tbls apple cider vinegar

- 1 Tbls honey

- 1 tsp Dijon mustard

- 1/3 cup extra virgin olive oil

- Salt and pepper to taste

Proc.: Preheat oven to 425°F (220°C)

- Toss sweet potato cubes with olive oil, salt, and pepper on a baking sheet

- Roast for 25 minutes, stirring halfway, until tender and caramelized

- Whisk together apple cider vinegar, honey, Dijon mustard, extra virgin olive oil, salt, and pepper to create the dressing

- In a large bowl, combine the roasted sweet potatoes, kale, dried cranberries, and walnuts

- Drizzle with the dressing and toss to coat evenly

- Serve immediately or let sit for the flavors to meld

N.V.: Calories: 320, Fat: 20g, Carbs: 33g, Protein: 5g, Sugar: 12g

CHICKPEA AND TUNA SALAD WITH LEMON VINAIGRETTE

P.T.: 15 min | **C.T.:** 0 min

M. of C.: No Cooking | **Serves:** 4

Ingr.: 2 C. chickpeas, cooked and drained

- 2 cans tuna in water, drained and flaked

- 1 red bell pepper, diced

- ½ red onion, finely chopped

- ¼ C. Kalamata olives, pitted and halved

- 2 Tbls capers

- ¼ C. parsley, chopped

- For the dressing: 3 Tbls extra virgin olive oil

- 1 Tbls lemon juice

- 1 tsp Dijon mustard

- 1 clove garlic, minced

- Salt and pepper to taste

Proc.: Whisk together dressing ingredients in a bowl

- In a large mixing bowl, combine chickpeas, tuna, red bell pepper, red onion, olives, capers, and parsley

- Pour dressing over the salad and toss to evenly coat

- Refrigerate before serving

N.V.: Calories: 330, Fat: 15g, Carbs: 23g, Protein: 25g, Sugar: 4g

QUINOA AND BLACK BEAN SALAD WITH AVOCADO

P.T.: 20 min | **C.T.:** 0 min

M. of C.: No Cooking | **Serves:** 4

Ingr.: 1 C. quinoa, cooked and cooled

- 1 C. black beans, cooked and drained

- 1 avocado, diced

- 1 mango, diced

- ½ C. cucumber, diced

- ¼ C. red onion, finely chopped

- ¼ C. cilantro, chopped

- For the dressing: 2 Tbls lime juice

- 1 Tbls extra virgin olive oil

- 1 tsp honey

- 1 clove garlic, minced

- 1 tsp cumin

- Salt and pepper to taste

Proc.: In a small bowl, whisk together dressing ingredients

- In a larger bowl, mix quinoa, black beans, avocado, mango, cucumber, red onion, and cilantro

- Drizzle dressing over the salad and gently toss to combine

- Chill in the refrigerator before serving

N.V.: Calories: 310, Fat: 10g, Carbs: 45g, Protein: 10g, Sugar: 8g

GREEK CHICKEN SALAD WITH HERB DRESSING

P.T.: 25 min | **C.T.:** 15 min

M. of C.: Grilling | **Serves:** 4

Ingr.: 2 C. chicken breast, grilled and sliced

- 3 C. Romaine lettuce, chopped

- 1 C. cherry tomatoes, halved

- ½ C. cucumber, sliced

- ¼ C. red onion, thinly sliced

- ½ C. feta cheese, crumbled

- ¼ C. olives, pitted

- For the dressing: 3 Tbls olive oil

- 1 Tbls red wine vinegar

- 1 tsp oregano, dried

- 1 clove garlic, minced

- Salt and pepper to taste

Proc.: Whisk together dressing ingredients in a bowl

- In a large salad bowl, combine lettuce, cherry tomatoes, cucumber, red onion, olives, and crumbled feta

- Top with grilled chicken slices

- Pour dressing over the salad and toss gently to combine

N.V.: Calories: 350, Fat: 18g, Carbs: 12g, Protein: 35g, Sugar: 3g

CHICKPEA AND QUINOA POWER SALAD

P.T.: 15 min | **C.T.:** 0 min

M. of C.: Mixing | **Serves:** 4

Ingr.: 1 cup quinoa, cooked and cooled

- 1 can (15 oz.) chickpeas, rinsed and drained

- 1 cucumber, diced

- 1 red bell pepper, diced

- 1/4 cup red onion, finely chopped

- 1/4 cup parsley, chopped

- For the dressing: 3 Tbls olive oil

- 2 Tbls lemon juice

- 1 tsp Dijon mustard

- 1 garlic clove, minced

- Salt and pepper to taste

- 1/4 cup feta cheese, crumbled (optional)

Proc.: In a large bowl, combine cooked quinoa, chickpeas, cucumber, red bell pepper, red onion, and parsley

- In a small bowl, whisk together olive oil, lemon juice, Dijon mustard, minced garlic, salt, and pepper to create the dressing

- Pour the dressing over the salad and toss to combine thoroughly

- Sprinkle with crumbled feta cheese before serving

N.V.: Calories: 330, Fat: 14g, Carbs: 42g, Protein: 12g, Sugar: 5g

4.3 DRESSINGS AND DIPS

AVOCADO CILANTRO LIME DRESSING

P.T.: 5 min | **C.T.:** 0 min

M. of C.: Blending | **Serves:** 8

Ingr.: 1 ripe avocado

- ¼ C. cilantro, fresh

- 2 Tbls lime juice

- 1 clove garlic

- ¼ C. Greek yogurt, plain

- 2 Tbls olive oil

- 1 Tbls water, or more as needed

- Salt and pepper to taste

Proc.: Combine avocado, cilantro, lime juice, garlic, Greek yogurt, and olive oil in a blender

- Blend until smooth, adding water as needed to reach desired consistency

- Season with salt and pepper to taste

- Serve immediately or store in the fridge

N.V.: Calories: 60, Fat: 5g, Carbs: 3g, Protein: 1g, Sugar: 1g

TAHINI GINGER DRESSING

P.T.: 5 min | **C.T.:** 0 min

M. of C.: Whisking | **Serves:** 8

Ingr.: ¼ C. tahini

- 2 Tbls soy sauce

- 1 Tbls apple cider vinegar

- 1 Tbls maple syrup

- 1 tsp ginger, grated

- 2 tsp sesame oil

- 3 Tbls water, or more for thinning

- 1 tsp garlic, minced

Proc.: In a bowl, whisk together tahini, soy sauce, apple cider vinegar, maple syrup, ginger, sesame oil, and garlic

- Gradually add water until desired consistency is achieved

- Adjust seasoning if necessary

- Use immediately or store in the refrigerator

N.V.: Calories: 80, Fat: 6g, Carbs: 6g, Protein: 2g, Sugar: 3g

CREAMY DILL AND YOGURT DIP

P.T.: 10 min | **C.T.:** 0 min

M. of C.: Mixing | **Serves:** 6

Ingr.: 1 C. Greek yogurt, plain

- 2 Tbls dill, fresh, chopped

- 1 Tbls lemon juice

- 1 clove garlic, minced

- Salt and pepper to taste

- 1 tsp onion powder

- 1 Tbls cucumber, finely grated and drained

Proc.: In a medium bowl, combine Greek yogurt, chopped dill, lemon juice, minced garlic, salt, pepper, onion powder, and grated cucumber

- Mix well until all ingredients are fully incorporated

- Chill in the refrigerator for at least 30 minutes before serving to allow flavors to meld

N.V.: Calories: 45, Fat: 1g, Carbs: 4g, Protein: 6g, Sugar: 3g

ROASTED RED PEPPER & WALNUT DIP

P.T.: 15 min | **C.T.:** 0 min

M. of C.: Blending | **Serves:** 8

Ingr.: 1 jar (16 oz.) roasted red peppers, drained

- 1 C. walnuts, toasted

- 1 Tbls pomegranate molasses

- 2 Tbls olive oil

- 1 tsp smoked paprika

- ½ tsp cumin

- 1 garlic clove, minced

- Salt and pepper to taste

Proc.: Place all ingredients in a blender or food processor and blend until smooth

- Taste and adjust seasoning as needed, adding more salt or pepper if desired

- Chill in the refrigerator for at least 1 hr before serving to allow flavors to meld

N.V.: Calories: 140, Fat: 12g, Carbs: 6g, Protein: 3g, Sugar: 2g

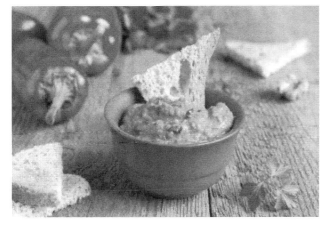

CHAPTER 5: FISH AND SEAFOOD RECIPES

Diving into the deep, refreshing waters of nutrition, Chapter 4 opens up a world where the bounty of the sea meets the art of anti-inflammatory eating. Fish and seafood are not just sources of high-quality protein; they are treasure troves of omega-3 fatty acids, essential for reducing inflammation and supporting heart and brain health. This chapter is dedicated to exploring the rich flavors and immense health benefits that fish and seafood can bring to our tables.

From the simplicity of grilled fish, kissed by smoke and flame, to the comfort of hearty seafood stews brimming with nourishment, we journey through recipes designed to suit every palate and occasion. Whether you're looking to impress guests with a light and refreshing seafood salad or seeking the solace of a baked salmon on a quiet evening, this collection promises to enhance your culinary repertoire with dishes that are as beneficial as they are delicious.

With a focus on sustainability and seasonality, we highlight ways to choose the best fish and seafood, ensuring that every bite contributes not only to our health but also to the health of our oceans. The recipes in this chapter are crafted to be accessible, guiding you through a variety of cooking techniques and flavor profiles, from the Mediterranean's citrusy zests to the bold spices of Asian cuisine.

As we navigate these waters together, let this chapter be your compass, leading you to meals that are both nourishing and delightful. Embark on this flavorful voyage with us, where every recipe is a step closer to a healthier, more vibrant you.

5.1 SIMPLE GRILLED AND BAKED FISH

LEMON HERB BAKED SALMON

P.T.: 10 min | **C.T.:** 20 min

M. of C.: Baking | **Serves:** 4

Ingr.: 4 salmon fillets, 6 oz each

- 2 Tbls olive oil

- 1 lemon, thinly sliced

- 2 garlic cloves, minced

- 1 tsp dried oregano

- 1 tsp dried thyme

- Salt and pepper to taste

Proc.: Preheat oven to 375°F (190°C)

- Arrange salmon fillets on a baking sheet lined with parchment paper

- Drizzle with olive oil and season with garlic, oregano, thyme, salt, and pepper

- Top each fillet with lemon slices

- Bake for 20 min or until salmon is flaky and opaque

- Serve immediately

N.V.: Calories: 280, Fat: 18g, Carbs: 2g, Protein: 26g, Sugar: 0g

SIMPLE GRILLED TILAPIA WITH AVOCADO SALSA

P.T.: 15 min | **C.T.:** 10 min

M. of C.: Grilling | **Serves:** 4

Ingr.: 4 tilapia fillets, 6 oz each

- 1 Tbls olive oil

- 1 avocado, diced

- 1 tomato, diced

- ¼ C. red onion, finely chopped

- 2 Tbls cilantro, chopped

- Juice of 1 lime

- Salt and pepper to taste

Proc.: Preheat grill to medium-high heat

- Brush tilapia fillets with olive oil and season with salt and pepper

- Grill for 4-5 minutes on each side or until fish flakes easily with a fork

- In a bowl, mix avocado, tomato, red onion, cilantro, lime juice, salt, and pepper to make the salsa

- Top grilled tilapia with avocado salsa and serve immediately

N.V.: Calories: 230, Fat: 12g, Carbs: 6g, Protein: 26g, Sugar: 2g

OVEN-ROASTED COD WITH CHERRY TOMATOES

P.T.: 10 min | **C.T.:** 15 min

M. of C.: Roasting | **Serves:** 4

Ingr.: 4 cod fillets, 6 oz each

- 2 C. cherry tomatoes

- 1 Tbls capers

- 3 Tbls olive oil

- 2 garlic cloves, minced

- 1 tsp balsamic vinegar

- Salt and pepper to taste

- Fresh basil leaves for garnish

Proc.: Preheat oven to 400°F (200°C)

- Place cod fillets in a baking dish

- In a bowl, toss cherry tomatoes, capers, olive oil, garlic, balsamic vinegar, salt, and pepper

- Pour mixture over cod and bake for 15 min or until cod is cooked through

- Garnish with fresh basil leaves before serving

N.V.: Calories: 220, Fat: 10g, Carbs: 6g, Protein: 27g, Sugar: 3g

PESTO-STUFFED TROUT

P.T.: 20 min | **C.T.:** 25 min

M. of C.: Baking | **Serves:** 4

Ingr.: 4 whole trout, cleaned and gutted

- ½ C. basil pesto

- 2 tomatoes, thinly sliced

- 2 lemons, thinly sliced

- 4 garlic cloves, thinly sliced

- Salt and pepper to taste

- Olive oil for drizzling

Proc.: Preheat oven to 375°F (190°C)

- Season the inside of each trout with salt and pepper

- Spread basil pesto inside each trout

- Layer tomato slices, lemon slices, and garlic slices inside the fish

- Drizzle with olive oil and season the outside with salt and pepper

- Bake for 25 min or until fish is cooked through and flaky

- Serve immediately

N.V.: Calories: 310, Fat: 20g, Carbs: 6g, Protein: 28g, Sugar: 2g

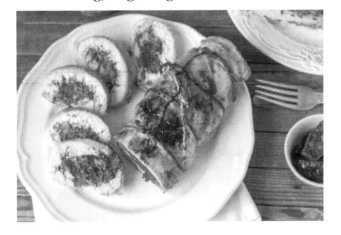

LEMON-HERB BAKED SALMON

P.T.: 10 min | **C.T.:** 20 min

M. of C.: Baking | **Serves:** 4

Ingr.: 4 salmon fillets, skin on

- 2 Tbls olive oil

- Juice and zest of 1 lemon

- 2 cloves garlic, minced

- 1 tsp dried oregano

- 1 tsp dried thyme

- Salt and pepper to taste

- 1 lemon, sliced for garnish

- Fresh dill for garnish

Proc.: Preheat oven to 400°F (200°C)

- In a small bowl, mix olive oil, lemon juice and zest, garlic, oregano, thyme, salt, and pepper

- Place salmon fillets skin-side down on a baking sheet lined with parchment paper

- Brush the lemon-herb mixture over the salmon fillets

- Bake for 20 minutes, or until salmon flakes easily with a fork

- Garnish with lemon slices and fresh dill before serving

N.V.: Calories: 280, Fat: 18g, Carbs: 2g, Protein: 25g, Sugar: 1g

5.2 HEARTY SEAFOOD STEWS AND SOUPS

SAFFRON SEAFOOD CHOWDER

P.T.: 20 min | **C.T.:** 40 min

M. of C.: Simmering | **Serves:** 6

Ingr.: 1 Tbls olive oil

- 1 onion, diced

- 2 garlic cloves, minced

- 2 carrots, diced

- 2 stalks celery, diced

- 1 lb. potatoes, cubed

- 1 quart vegetable broth

- 1 pinch saffron threads

- 1 lb. mixed seafood (shrimp, scallops, and firm white fish), chopped

- 1 C. coconut milk

- Salt and pepper to taste

- Fresh parsley, chopped for garnish

Proc.: Heat olive oil in a large pot over medium heat

- Sauté onion and garlic until soft

- Add carrots, celery, and potatoes, cook for 5 min

- Pour in vegetable broth and bring to a boil

- Add saffron, reduce heat, and simmer for 20 min or until vegetables are tender

- Add seafood and cook for an additional 10 min or until seafood is cooked through

- Stir in coconut milk, season with salt and pepper, and heat through

- Serve garnished with fresh parsley

N.V.: Calories: 250, Fat: 8g, Carbs: 25g, Protein: 20g, Sugar: 5g

TOMATO BASIL SHRIMP STEW

P.T.: 15 min | **C.T.:** 25 min

M. of C.: Simmering | **Serves:** 4

Ingr.: 2 Tbls extra virgin olive oil

- 1 lb. shrimp, peeled and deveined

- 1 onion, chopped

- 3 garlic cloves, minced

- 1 can (28 oz.) diced tomatoes

- 2 cups vegetable broth

- 1 tsp dried basil

- 1 tsp dried oregano

- Salt and pepper to taste

- ½ C. fresh basil, torn

- Grated Parmesan cheese for serving

Proc.: Heat olive oil in a large pot over medium heat

- Add shrimp and cook until pink, set aside

- In the same pot, add onion and garlic, cook until translucent

- Pour in diced tomatoes and vegetable broth, bring to a simmer

- Add dried basil and oregano, season with salt and pepper

- Return shrimp to the pot, simmer for 15 min

- Stir in fresh basil just before serving

- Serve with grated Parmesan cheese on top

N.V.: Calories: 230, Fat: 8g, Carbs: 14g, Protein: 25g, Sugar: 6g

LEMONGRASS MUSSELS SOUP

P.T.: 10 min | **C.T.:** 15 min

M. of C.: Boiling | **Serves:** 4

Ingr.: 2 stalks lemongrass, minced

- 1 inch ginger, minced

- 1 lb. mussels, cleaned

- 1 can (13.5 oz) coconut milk

- 2 cups vegetable broth

- 1 Tbls fish sauce

- 1 tsp sugar

- 2 green onions, sliced

- 1 Tbls lime juice

- Fresh cilantro for garnish

Proc.: In a large pot, bring lemongrass, ginger, coconut milk, and vegetable broth to a boil

- Add mussels, cover, and cook until they open, about 5-7 min

- Stir in fish sauce, sugar, and lime juice

- Serve garnished with green onions and fresh cilantro

N.V.: Calories: 200, Fat: 12g, Carbs: 10g, Protein: 14g, Sugar: 3g

MEDITERRANEAN SEAFOOD STEW

P.T.: 15 min | **C.T.:** 45 min

M. of C.: Simmering | **Serves:** 6

Ingr.: 1 lb mixed seafood (shrimp, scallops, and firm white fish like cod), cleaned and cut into pieces

- 2 Tbls olive oil

- 1 onion, chopped

- 2 cloves garlic, minced

- 1 bell pepper, diced

- 1 can (14 oz) diced tomatoes

- 2 cups fish or vegetable broth

- 1 cup white wine

- 1 tsp dried oregano

- 1 tsp dried basil

- 1/2 tsp red pepper flakes

- Salt and pepper to taste

- 1/4 cup fresh parsley, chopped

- Juice of 1 lemon

Proc.: Heat olive oil in a large pot over medium heat

- Sauté onion, garlic, and bell pepper until softened

- Add diced tomatoes, broth, white wine, oregano, basil, red pepper flakes, salt, and pepper

- Bring to a boil, then reduce heat and simmer for 30 minutes

- Add the mixed seafood and simmer for an additional 10-15 minutes, or until seafood is cooked through

- Stir in fresh parsley and lemon juice just before serving

N.V.: Calories: 220, Fat: 8g, Carbs: 10g, Protein: 25g, Sugar: 4g

CITRUS SHRIMP AND AVOCADO SALAD

P.T.: 15 min | **C.T.:** 0 min

M. of C.: No Cooking | **Serves:** 4

Ingr.: 1 lb. shrimp, cooked and peeled

- 2 avocados, diced

- 1 grapefruit, segmented

- 1 orange, segmented

- ½ red onion, thinly sliced

- ¼ C. cilantro, chopped

- For the dressing: 2 Tbls olive oil

- 1 Tbls lime juice

- 1 tsp honey

- Salt and pepper to taste

Proc.: In a large bowl, combine shrimp, avocados, grapefruit segments, orange segments, red onion, and cilantro

- Whisk together olive oil, lime juice, honey, salt, and pepper to make the dressing

- Drizzle dressing over the salad and gently toss to combine

- Serve immediately

N.V.: Calories: 290, Fat: 18g, Carbs: 20g, Protein: 17g, Sugar: 10g

ASIAN CRAB AND CUCUMBER SALAD

P.T.: 20 min | **C.T.:** 0 min

M. of C.: No Cooking | **Serves:** 4

Ingr.: 1 lb. crabmeat, fresh or canned and drained

- 2 cucumbers, spiralized or thinly sliced

- 1 carrot, julienned

- ½ C. radishes, thinly sliced

- ¼ C. green onions, chopped

- For the dressing: 3 Tbls soy sauce

- 1 Tbls sesame oil

- 2 tsp rice vinegar

- 1 tsp honey

- 1 garlic clove, minced

- 1 Tbls ginger, grated

- Sesame seeds for garnish

Proc.: In a large bowl, mix together crabmeat, cucumbers, carrot, radishes, and green onions

- Whisk together soy sauce, sesame oil, rice vinegar, honey, garlic, and ginger to create the dressing

- Pour dressing over the salad and toss to evenly coat

- Garnish with sesame seeds before serving

N.V.: Calories: 180, Fat: 7g, Carbs: 12g, Protein: 16g, Sugar: 6g

MEDITERRANEAN OCTOPUS SALAD

P.T.: 30 min | **C.T.:** 1 hr

M. of C.: Boiling and Cooling | **Serves:** 4

Ingr.: 1 lb. octopus, cleaned

- 1 lemon, halved

- 1 bay leaf

- 2 C. cherry tomatoes, halved

- 1 C. cucumber, diced

- ½ C. Kalamata olives, pitted

- ¼ C. red onion, thinly sliced

- ¼ C. parsley, chopped

- For the dressing: 3 Tbls extra virgin olive oil

- 1 Tbls red wine vinegar

- 1 tsp oregano, dried

- Salt and pepper to taste

Proc.: In a large pot, combine octopus, lemon halves, and bay leaf with water to cover

- Bring to a boil, then reduce heat and simmer for 45-60 min or until octopus is tender

- Remove octopus, let cool, then cut into bite-size pieces

- Combine octopus with tomatoes, cucumber, olives, red onion, and parsley in a salad bowl

- Mix olive oil, red wine vinegar, oregano, salt, and pepper to make the dressing

- Pour dressing over salad and toss well to coat

- Serve chilled or at room temperature

N.V.: Calories: 250, Fat: 14g, Carbs: 15g, Protein: 20g, Sugar: 4g

SEARED SCALLOP AND GRAPEFRUIT SALAD

P.T.: 20 min | **C.T.:** 10 min

M. of C.: Searing | **Serves:** 4

Ingr.: 12 sea scallops, patted dry

- 1 Tbls avocado oil

- 2 grapefruits, one juiced and one segmented

- 1 avocado, sliced

- 4 cups arugula

- 1/4 cup thinly sliced red onion

- 1 Tbls honey

- 2 Tbls extra virgin olive oil

- 1 tsp Dijon mustard

- Salt and black pepper to taste

Proc.: Season scallops with salt and pepper

- Heat avocado oil in a pan over medium-high heat and sear scallops for about 2 min on each side until a golden crust forms

- Whisk together grapefruit juice, honey, extra virgin olive oil, Dijon mustard, salt, and pepper to make the dressing

- Toss arugula, grapefruit segments, sliced avocado, and red onion with the dressing

- Top the salad with seared scallops and serve immediately

N.V.: Calories: 290, Fat: 15g, Carbs: 22g, Protein: 19g, Sugar: 12g

CHAPTER 6: POULTRY RECIPES

In the heart of every home kitchen lies the comforting and versatile ingredient: poultry. Chapter 5 of our culinary journey introduces an array of delightful poultry recipes, each infused with anti-inflammatory ingredients to nourish your body and soul. Poultry, a lean protein source, is not only a cornerstone of a balanced diet but also pairs wonderfully with a spectrum of flavors and ingredients that combat inflammation.

This chapter is dedicated to reimagining chicken and turkey beyond their traditional roles. From the sizzle of stir-fries brimming with colorful vegetables to the soothing warmth of broths and stews, these recipes are designed to bring variety and excitement to your table. We explore innovative baking and roasting techniques that lock in flavors and nutrients, ensuring every bite is a step toward wellness.

Our poultry dishes are more than just meals; they are a means of gathering, sharing, and taking care of our health. With ingredients like turmeric, ginger, and garlic, we harness the power of nature's anti-inflammatory gifts. Each recipe is crafted to be straightforward and adaptable, catering to the busy lives we lead without compromising on taste or nutritional value.

As we venture through the recipes in this chapter, let's embrace the simplicity and richness poultry offers. Whether you're seeking comfort food with an anti-inflammatory twist or light and refreshing meals, there's something here for every occasion. Let these recipes inspire you to create dishes that are both healing and heartwarming, turning everyday meals into opportunities for well-being.

6.1 FLAVORFUL CHICKEN AND TURKEY STIR-FRIES

GINGER-TURMERIC CHICKEN STIR-FRY

P.T.: 15 min | **C.T.:** 10 min

M. of C.: Stir-Frying |

Serves: 4

Ingr.: 1 lb. chicken breast, thinly sliced

- 2 Tbls coconut oil

- 1 red bell pepper, julienned

- 1 C. broccoli florets

- ½ C. snap peas

- 1 carrot, julienned

- For the sauce: 2 Tbls soy sauce

- 1 Tbls honey

- 1 Tbls freshly grated ginger

- 1 tsp ground turmeric

- 2 garlic cloves, minced

- 1 tsp sesame oil

- Salt and pepper to taste

Proc.: Heat coconut oil in a large pan over medium-high heat

- Add chicken and stir-fry until browned

- Add vegetables and stir-fry for an additional 5 minutes

- Whisk together sauce ingredients and pour over chicken and vegetables

- Cook for 2-3 minutes, until sauce thickens and vegetables are tender but crisp

- Serve immediately

N.V.: Calories: 250, Fat: 10g, Carbs: 15g, Protein: 26g, Sugar: 7g

LEMONY BASIL TURKEY STIR-FRY

P.T.: 10 min | **C.T.:** 12 min

M. of C.: Stir-Frying | **Serves:** 4

Ingr.: 1 lb. turkey breast, thinly sliced

- 2 Tbls olive oil

- 1 zucchini, sliced

- 1 yellow squash, sliced

- 1 red onion, sliced

- For the sauce: Juice of 1 lemon

- 2 Tbls soy sauce

- 1 Tbls honey

- 1 cup fresh basil leaves, chopped

- 2 garlic cloves, minced

- Salt and pepper to taste

Proc.: Heat olive oil in a skillet over medium-high heat

- Add turkey and stir-fry until no longer pink

- Add zucchini, squash, and onion, and stir-fry for 5-7 minutes until vegetables are tender

- Mix sauce ingredients and pour over the turkey and vegetables

- Stir well to combine and cook for an additional 2 minutes

- Serve hot

N.V.: Calories: 220, Fat: 8g, Carbs: 12g, Protein: 29g, Sugar: 6g

SPICY SZECHUAN CHICKEN STIR-FRY

P.T.: 20 min | **C.T.:** 15 min

M. of C.: Stir-Frying | **Serves:** 4

Ingr.: 1 lb. chicken thighs, cut into bite-sized pieces

- 2 Tbls peanut oil

- 1 bell pepper, cut into strips

- ½ C. dry roasted peanuts

- 4 green onions, chopped

- For the sauce: 2 Tbls hoisin sauce

- 1 Tbls soy sauce

- 1 Tbls rice vinegar

- 1 tsp chili paste

- 1 Tbls honey

- 2 garlic cloves, minced

- 1 tsp grated ginger

- 1 tsp sesame oil

- Salt to taste

Proc.: Heat peanut oil in a wok over high heat

- Add chicken and stir-fry until browned

- Add bell pepper and stir-fry for 3 minutes

- Lower heat to medium, add peanuts and green onions

- Whisk together sauce ingredients and pour over the chicken mixture

- Stir well to coat and cook until the sauce is heated through

- Serve with steamed jasmine rice

N.V.: Calories: 320, Fat: 18g, Carbs: 15g, Protein: 28g, Sugar: 8g

THAI BASIL CHICKEN STIR-FRY

P.T.: 15 min | **C.T.:** 10 min

M. of C.: Stir-Frying | **Serves:** 4

Ingr.: 1 lb. ground chicken

- 2 Tbls vegetable oil

- 3 cloves garlic, minced

- 1 red chili, finely sliced

- 2 shallots, thinly sliced

- 1 bell pepper, diced

- For the sauce: 2 Tbls fish sauce

- 1 Tbls soy sauce

- 1 Tbls oyster sauce

- 1 tsp sugar

- 1 C. Thai basil leaves

Proc.: Heat oil in a large pan over medium-high heat

- Add garlic, chili, and shallots, stir-frying until fragrant

- Add ground chicken, breaking it apart and cook until browned

- Add bell pepper and stir-fry for 2 minutes

- Mix in sauce ingredients, then fold in Thai basil leaves until wilted

- Remove from heat and serve immediately

N.V.: Calories: 270, Fat: 15g, Carbs: 8g, Protein: 27g, Sugar: 4g

TURMERIC CHICKEN AND BROCCOLI STIR-FRY

P.T.: 15 min | **C.T.:** 20 min

M. of C.: Stir-Frying | **Serves:** 4

Ingr.: 1 lb chicken breast, thinly sliced

- 2 Tbls coconut oil

- 1 head of broccoli, cut into florets

- 1 red bell pepper, sliced

- 1 yellow bell pepper, sliced

- 2 cloves garlic, minced

- 1 Tbls fresh ginger, grated

- 1 tsp turmeric powder

- 2 Tbls soy sauce (or tamari for gluten-free option)

- 1 tsp honey

- Juice of 1 lime

- Salt and pepper to taste

- 1/4 cup cilantro, chopped for garnish

Proc.: Heat coconut oil in a large skillet or wok over medium-high heat

- Add chicken slices, seasoning with salt and pepper, and stir-fry until browned and cooked through

- Remove chicken and set aside

- In the same skillet, add more coconut oil if needed, then stir-fry broccoli and bell peppers until tender-crisp

- Add garlic, ginger, and turmeric, stirring frequently for about 1 minute

- Return chicken to the skillet, add soy sauce, honey, and lime juice, tossing everything to combine well

- Cook for an additional 2-3 minutes

6.2 COMFORTING SOUPS AND STEWS

CREAMY CHICKEN AND MUSHROOM SOUP

P.T.: 10 min | **C.T.:** 30 min

M. of C.: Simmering | **Serves:** 4

Ingr.: 1 lb. chicken breast, cubed

- 1 Tbls olive oil

- 1 onion, diced

- 2 garlic cloves, minced

- 8 oz. mushrooms, sliced

- 4 cups chicken broth

- 1 cup coconut milk

- 1 tsp thyme

- 1 tsp rosemary

- Salt and pepper to taste

- 2 Tbls arrowroot powder mixed with 2 Tbls water

Proc.: Heat olive oil in a large pot over medium heat

- Sauté onion and garlic until translucent

- Add chicken and cook until browned

- Add mushrooms and sauté for 5 minutes

- Pour in chicken broth and bring to a simmer

- Add thyme, rosemary, salt, and pepper

- Stir in coconut milk and arrowroot mixture to thicken

- Serve garnished with chopped cilantro

N.V.: Calories: 240, Fat: 9g, Carbs: 15g, Protein: 27g, Sugar: 5g

- Simmer for 20 minutes

- Serve hot

N.V.: Calories: 240, Fat: 12g, Carbs: 10g, Protein: 22g, Sugar: 4g

TURKEY AND SWEET POTATO STEW

P.T.: 15 min | **C.T.:** 40 min

M. of C.: Boiling | **Serves:** 6

Ingr.: 1 lb. ground turkey

- 1 Tbls coconut oil

- 1 onion, chopped

- 2 carrots, diced

- 2 sweet potatoes, cubed

- 4 cups chicken broth

- 1 can (14.5 oz) diced tomatoes

- 1 tsp paprika

- 1 tsp cumin

- Salt and pepper to taste

- 2 cups spinach, roughly chopped

Proc.: Heat coconut oil in a large pot over medium heat

- Cook turkey until browned

- Add onion, carrots, and sweet potatoes, cooking until slightly softened

- Pour in chicken broth and diced tomatoes

- Season with paprika, cumin, salt, and pepper
- Bring to a boil, then simmer for 30 minutes or until sweet potatoes are tender
- Stir in spinach just before serving and cook until wilted
- Serve warm

N.V.: Calories: 260, Fat: 8g, Carbs: 25g, Protein: 20g, Sugar: 7g

LEMONGRASS CHICKEN SOUP

P.T.: 20 min | **C.T.:** 25 min

M. of C.: Simmering | **Serves:** 4

Ingr.: 1 lb. chicken thighs, sliced

- 1 Tbls sesame oil
- 4 cups chicken broth
- 1 stalk lemongrass, minced
- 1 inch ginger, sliced
- 2 carrots, sliced
- 1 bell pepper, julienned
- 1 cup mushrooms, sliced
- 2 Tbls fish sauce
- Juice of 1 lime
- Salt to taste
- Fresh cilantro for garnish

Proc.: Heat sesame oil in a large pot over medium heat

- Add chicken and cook until no longer pink
- Pour in chicken broth and add lemongrass and ginger
- Bring to a simmer

- Add carrots, bell pepper, and mushrooms, cooking until vegetables are tender
- Stir in fish sauce and lime juice, adjusting salt to taste
- Garnish with fresh cilantro before serving

N.V.: Calories: 220, Fat: 9g, Carbs: 10g, Protein: 26g, Sugar: 5g

LEMON CHICKEN ORZO SOUP

P.T.: 10 min | **C.T.:** 30 min

M. of C.: Simmering | **Serves:** 6

Ingr.: 1 Tbls olive oil

- 1 lb chicken breasts
- Salt and pepper to taste
- 1 onion, diced
- 2 carrots, peeled and diced
- 2 celery stalks, diced
- 3 cloves garlic, minced
- 6 cups chicken broth
- Juice and zest of 2 lemons
- 1 tsp dried thyme
- 1 cup orzo pasta
- 2 cups spinach, roughly chopped
- 1/4 cup fresh parsley, chopped

Proc.: Heat olive oil in a large pot over medium heat

- Season chicken breasts with salt and pepper, add to the pot, and cook until golden and cooked through, about 5-7 minutes per side
- Remove chicken, let it cool, then shred

- In the same pot, add onion, carrots, and celery, and sauté until softened

- Stir in garlic and cook for another minute

- Pour in chicken broth, lemon juice, and zest, then bring to a simmer

- Add thyme and orzo, cooking until orzo is tender, about 10 minutes

- Return shredded chicken to the pot, add spinach and parsley, and cook until the spinach is wilted

- Season with salt and pepper to taste before serving

next day as the flavors meld together

N.V.: Calories: 220, Fat: 4g, Carbs: 25g, Protein: 20g, Sugar: 3g

6.3 HEALTHY BAKED AND ROASTED OPTIONS

TURMERIC ROASTED CHICKEN WITH VEGETABLES

P.T.: 15 min | **C.T.:** 1 hr

M. of C.: Roasting | **Serves:** 4

Ingr.: 1 whole chicken, about 4 lbs

- 2 Tbls olive oil

- 1 tsp ground turmeric

- 1 tsp smoked paprika

- Salt and pepper to taste

- 4 carrots, cut into chunks

- 3 parsnips, cut into chunks

- 1 sweet potato, cubed

- 1 onion, quartered

- 4 garlic cloves, minced

Proc.: Preheat oven to 425°F (220°C)

- In a small bowl, mix olive oil, turmeric, paprika, salt, and pepper

- Rub the mixture all over the chicken

- Place chicken in a roasting pan and surround with carrots, parsnips, sweet potato, onion, and garlic

- Roast for 1 hour or until the chicken is cooked through and vegetables are tender

- Let chicken rest for 10 minutes before carving

N.V.: Calories: 450, Fat: 22g, Carbs: 30g, Protein: 35g, Sugar: 8g

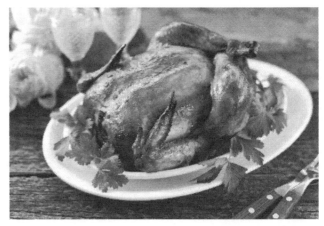

BALSAMIC GLAZED TURKEY BREAST

P.T.: 10 min | **C.T.:** 1 hr 30 min

M. of C.: Baking | **Serves:** 6

Ingr.: 1 turkey breast (3 lbs)

- ¼ cup balsamic vinegar

- 2 Tbls honey

- 1 Tbls Dijon mustard

- 2 garlic cloves, minced

- 1 tsp rosemary, chopped

- Salt and pepper to taste

- 1 Tbls olive oil

Proc.: Preheat oven to 350°F (175°C)

- In a bowl, whisk together balsamic vinegar, honey, Dijon mustard, garlic, rosemary, salt, and pepper

- Place turkey breast in a baking dish and brush with olive oil

- Generously apply the balsamic mixture over the turkey

- Bake for 1 hour and 30 minutes, basting every 30 minutes with pan juices, until cooked through

- Let rest for 10 minutes before slicing

N.V.: Calories: 320, Fat: 5g, Carbs: 12g, Protein: 55g, Sugar: 11g

LEMON GARLIC HERB ROASTED CHICKEN THIGHS

P.T.: 20 min | **C.T.:** 40 min

M. of C.: Roasting | **Serves:** 4

Ingr.: 8 chicken thighs, bone-in and skin-on

- 4 Tbls olive oil

- 2 lemons, 1 juiced and 1 sliced

- 4 garlic cloves, minced

- 1 Tbls thyme, chopped

- 1 Tbls rosemary, chopped

- Salt and pepper to taste

Proc.: Preheat oven to 400°F (200°C)

- In a large bowl, combine olive oil, lemon juice, minced garlic, thyme, rosemary, salt, and pepper

- Add chicken thighs and toss to coat thoroughly

- Arrange chicken in a single layer on a baking sheet and place lemon slices around chicken

- Roast for 40 minutes or until the skin is crispy and chicken is cooked through

- Serve hot, garnished with additional fresh herbs if desired

N.V.: Calories: 390, Fat: 28g, Carbs: 5g, Protein: 30g, Sugar: 1g

HERB-CRUSTED CHICKEN WITH ROASTED VEGETABLES

P.T.: 15 min | **C.T.:** 35 min

M. of C.: Roasting | **Serves:** 4

Ingr.: 4 boneless, skinless chicken breasts

- 1 Tbls olive oil

- 1 tsp rosemary, minced

- 1 tsp thyme, minced

- 1 tsp oregano, minced

- Salt and pepper to taste

- 2 cups Brussels sprouts, halved

- 1 cup carrots, sliced

- 1 cup parsnips, sliced

- 2 Tbls balsamic vinegar

- 1 Tbls honey

Proc.: Preheat oven to 425°F (220°C)

- In a small bowl, combine olive oil, rosemary, thyme, oregano, salt, and pepper

- Rub the herb mixture over the chicken breasts

- Arrange the chicken and vegetables on a large baking sheet

- Whisk together balsamic vinegar and honey, drizzle over the vegetables

- Roast in the oven for 35 minutes, or until the chicken is cooked through and the vegetables are tender and caramelized

N.V.: Calories: 320, Fat: 8g, Carbs: 24g, Protein: 35g, Sugar: 10g

CHAPTER 7: SIDE DISH RECIPES

As we continue our journey through *The Ultimate Anti-Inflammatory Cookbook*, we arrive at a chapter dedicated to the unsung heroes of the dining table: side dishes. These culinary accompaniments, far from being mere afterthoughts, are pivotal in creating balanced, nutritious, and complete meals. Chapter 6 is a celebration of these dishes, each crafted to complement your main courses while packing a powerful punch of anti-inflammatory benefits.

In this collection, we delve into the colorful world of vegetables, whole grains, and legumes, transforming them into vibrant, flavorful creations that stand tall next to any entrée. From the crunch of a fresh salad to the comfort of roasted root vegetables, and the wholesomeness of ancient grains, these recipes are designed to enhance your mealtime with textures and flavors that delight the senses.

Here, you'll discover side dishes that serve not just as accompaniments, but as showcases for the nutritional powerhouses that are essential to an anti-inflammatory diet. We explore innovative ways to incorporate leafy greens, utilize anti-inflammatory spices, and unlock the potential of fermented foods for gut health.

This chapter is an invitation to elevate your meals with sides that are as nourishing as they are delicious. Whether you're looking to round out a weeknight dinner or add a healthful touch to a festive spread, these recipes offer the versatility and vibrancy to match any occasion. Let's embrace the art of the side dish, where every bite is a step toward wellness.

7.1 NUTRIENT-DENSE VEGETABLE SIDES

ROASTED BRUSSELS SPROUTS WITH BALSAMIC REDUCTION

P.T.: 10 min | **C.T.:** 20 min

M. of C.: Roasting | **Serves:** 4

Ingr.: 1 lb. Brussels sprouts, halved

- 2 Tbls olive oil

- Salt and pepper to taste

- ¼ cup balsamic vinegar

- 1 Tbls honey

Proc.: Preheat oven to 400°F (200°C)

- Toss Brussels sprouts with olive oil, salt, and pepper and spread on a baking sheet

- Roast for 20 minutes, turning halfway through, until crisp and golden

- While sprouts are roasting, simmer balsamic vinegar and honey in a small saucepan over low heat until thickened

- Drizzle balsamic reduction over roasted Brussels sprouts before serving

N.V.: Calories: 120, Fat: 7g, Carbs: 13g, Protein: 3g, Sugar: 7g

GARLIC TURMERIC CAULIFLOWER STEAKS

P.T.: 5 min | **C.T.:** 25 min

M. of C.: Baking | **Serves:** 4

Ingr.: 1 large head cauliflower, sliced into ½ inch steaks

- 3 Tbls coconut oil, melted

- 2 garlic cloves, minced

- 1 tsp turmeric

- Salt and pepper to taste

- Fresh parsley, chopped for garnish

Proc.: Preheat oven to 425°F (220°C)

- In a bowl, mix coconut oil, garlic, turmeric, salt, and pepper

- Brush both sides of cauliflower steaks with the mixture

- Place on a baking sheet and roast for 25 minutes, flipping halfway through, until tender and golden

- Garnish with parsley before serving

N.V.: Calories: 110, Fat: 10g, Carbs: 6g, Protein: 2g, Sugar: 2g

SPICY ROASTED SWEET POTATOES

P.T.: 10 min | **C.T.:** 35 min

M. of C.: Roasting | **Serves:** 4

Ingr.: 2 large sweet potatoes, cubed

- 2 Tbls olive oil

- 1 tsp smoked paprika

- ½ tsp cayenne pepper

- ½ tsp garlic powder

- Salt and pepper to taste

Proc.: Preheat oven to 375°F (190°C)

- Toss sweet potatoes with olive oil, smoked paprika, cayenne pepper, garlic powder, salt, and pepper in a bowl

- Spread on a baking sheet and roast for 35 minutes, stirring occasionally, until tender and caramelized

- Serve hot

N.V.: Calories: 200, Fat: 7g, Carbs: 33g, Protein: 2g, Sugar: 7g

ZESTY LEMON GREEN BEANS

P.T.: 5 min | **C.T.:** 15 min

M. of C.: Sautéing | **Serves:** 4

Ingr.: 1 lb. green beans, trimmed

- 2 Tbls almond oil

- Zest and juice of 1 lemon

- 2 garlic cloves, minced

- Salt and pepper to taste

- Almond slices, toasted for garnish

Proc.: Heat almond oil in a large skillet over medium heat

- Add green beans and cook, stirring frequently, for about 10 minutes until they begin to soften

- Add garlic, lemon zest, and lemon juice, and season with salt and pepper

- Cook for an additional 5 minutes

- Garnish with toasted almond slices before serving

N.V.: Calories: 90, Fat: 5g, Carbs: 10g, Protein: 2g, Sugar: 4g

GARLIC ROASTED RAINBOW CARROTS

P.T.: 10 min | **C.T.:** 25 min

M. of C.: Roasting | **Serves:** 4

Ingr.: 1 lb rainbow carrots, peeled and trimmed

- 2 Tbls olive oil

- 4 cloves garlic, minced

- 1 tsp thyme, fresh

- Salt and pepper to taste

- 1 Tbls parsley, chopped for garnish

Proc.: Preheat oven to 425°F (220°C)

- In a large bowl, toss the carrots with olive oil, minced garlic, thyme, salt, and pepper until evenly coated

- Spread the carrots in a single layer on a baking sheet

- Roast for 25 minutes, or until carrots are tender and slightly caramelized, turning halfway through

- Garnish with chopped parsley before serving

N.V.: Calories: 120, Fat: 7g, Carbs: 14g, Protein: 1g, Sugar: 7g

7.2 WHOLE GRAINS AND LEGUMES

MOROCCAN SPICED QUINOA

P.T.: 5 min | **C.T.:** 20 min

M. of C.: Simmering | **Serves:** 4

Ingr.: 1 C. quinoa, rinsed

- 2 C. vegetable broth

- 1 tsp cumin

- ½ tsp cinnamon

- ¼ tsp allspice

- 1 carrot, diced

- ½ C. raisins

- Salt and pepper to taste

- ¼ C. almonds, toasted

- 2 Tbls fresh parsley, chopped

Proc.: In a saucepan, bring vegetable broth to a boil

- Add quinoa, cumin, cinnamon, allspice, carrot, and raisins

- Season with salt and pepper

- Reduce heat to low, cover, and simmer for 20 minutes or until liquid is absorbed

- Fluff with a fork, then stir in toasted almonds and fresh parsley before serving

N.V.: Calories: 220, Fat: 5g, Carbs: 40g, Protein: 6g, Sugar: 10g

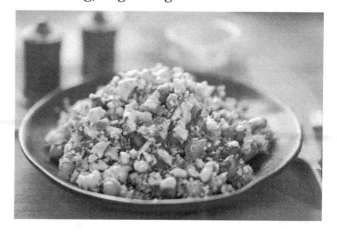

LEMONY LENTIL AND SPINACH SALAD

P.T.: 10 min | **C.T.:** 25 min

M. of C.: Boiling | **Serves:** 4

Ingr.: 1 C. green lentils, rinsed

- 4 C. water

- 1 bay leaf

- 2 C. spinach, chopped

- 1 red bell pepper, diced

- ¼ C. red onion, finely chopped

- For the dressing: 3 Tbls olive oil

- 2 Tbls lemon juice

- 1 garlic clove, minced

- 1 tsp Dijon mustard

- Salt and pepper to taste

Proc.: In a pot, combine lentils, water, and bay leaf

- Bring to a boil, then reduce heat and simmer for 25 minutes or until lentils are tender

- Discard bay leaf and drain lentils

- In a large bowl, combine warm lentils with spinach, bell pepper, and red onion

- Whisk together dressing ingredients and pour over the salad

- Toss to combine and serve warm or at room temperature

N.V.: Calories: 270, Fat: 10g, Carbs: 35g, Protein: 12g, Sugar: 3g

BARLEY AND MUSHROOM PILAF

P.T.: 15 min | **C.T.:** 45 min

M. of C.: Sautéing and Simmering

Serves: 6

Ingr.: 1 C. pearl barley, rinsed

- 2 Tbls olive oil

- 1 onion, diced

- 2 garlic cloves, minced

- 8 oz. mushrooms, sliced

- 3 C. vegetable broth

- 1 tsp thyme

- Salt and pepper to taste

- 2 Tbls fresh parsley, chopped

Proc.: Heat olive oil in a large skillet over medium heat

- Sauté onion and garlic until translucent

- Add mushrooms and cook until they begin to brown

- Stir in barley, vegetable broth, thyme, salt, and pepper

- Bring to a boil, then reduce heat, cover, and simmer for 45 minutes or until barley is tender and liquid is absorbed

- Stir in fresh parsley before serving

N.V.: Calories: 230, Fat: 7g, Carbs: 38g, Protein: 6g, Sugar: 2g

QUINOA TABBOULEH WITH CHICKPEAS

P.T.: 15 min | **C.T.:** 0 min

M. of C.: Mixing | **Serves:** 6

Ingr.: 2 cups quinoa, cooked and cooled

- 1 can (15 oz.) chickpeas, rinsed and drained

- 1 cucumber, diced

- 1 pint cherry tomatoes, halved

- 1/2 cup parsley, finely chopped

- 1/4 cup mint, finely chopped

- 3 Tbls olive oil

- Juice of 2 lemons

- 1 garlic clove, minced

- Salt and pepper to taste

Proc.: In a large bowl, combine cooked quinoa, chickpeas, cucumber, cherry tomatoes, parsley, and mint

- In a small bowl, whisk together olive oil, lemon juice, minced garlic, salt, and pepper to create the dressing

- Pour the dressing over the quinoa mixture and toss to combine thoroughly

- Adjust seasoning with salt and pepper as needed

- Serve chilled or at room temperature

N.V.: Calories: 220, Fat: 8g, Carbs: 32g, Protein: 8g, Sugar: 5g

HOMEMADE CLASSIC SAUERKRAUT

P.T.: 20 min | **C.T.:** 0 min

M. of C.: Fermenting | **Serves:** 8

Ingr.: 1 medium cabbage, finely shredded

- 1 Tbls sea salt

- 1 tsp caraway seeds (optional)

Proc.: In a large bowl, massage the shredded cabbage with sea salt until it starts to release liquid

- Continue to massage until there is enough liquid to cover the cabbage when pressed down

- Mix in caraway seeds if using

- Pack the mixture tightly into a clean jar, ensuring the cabbage is submerged under the liquid

- Cover the jar with a cloth and secure with a rubber band

- Let it sit at room temperature, away from direct sunlight, for at least 2 weeks, checking periodically to ensure cabbage remains submerged, until it reaches desired sourness

- Store in the refrigerator once fermentation is complete

N.V.: Calories: 27, Fat: 0g, Carbs: 6g, Protein: 1g, Sugar: 3g

QUICK KIMCHI

P.T.: 30 min | **C.T.:** 0 min

M. of C.: Fermenting | **Serves:** 6

Ingr.: 1 medium Napa cabbage, cut into 2-inch pieces

- ¼ cup sea salt

- Water

- 2 Tbls grated ginger

- 4 cloves garlic, minced

- 2 tsp sugar

- 3 Tbls fish sauce

- 1 Tbls soy sauce

- ½ cup Korean red pepper flakes (gochugaru)

- 1 daikon radish, julienned

- 4 green onions, cut into 1-inch pieces

Proc.: Place cabbage in a large bowl, sprinkle with sea salt, and cover with water

- Let stand for 2 hours, then rinse and drain

- In a separate bowl, mix ginger, garlic, sugar, fish sauce, soy sauce, and gochugaru to make the paste

- Add radish and green onions to the paste

- Mix in the drained cabbage until well coated

- Pack the mixture into a clean jar, pressing down to reduce air pockets and ensure the vegetables are submerged under the brine

- Cover loosely and let it ferment at room temperature for 2-5 days, checking daily to press down vegetables to keep them submerged

- Refrigerate after desired fermentation is reached

N.V.: Calories: 35, Fat: 0g, Carbs: 7g, Protein: 2g, Sugar: 4g

BEET KVASS

P.T.: 10 min | C.T.: 0 min

M. of C.: Fermenting | Serves: 4

Ingr.: 4 medium beets, cubed

- ¼ cup whey or an additional 1 Tbls sea salt if dairy-free

- 1 Tbls sea salt

- Water to fill a quart-sized jar

Proc.: Place beets in a clean quart-sized jar

- Add whey (if using) and sea salt

- Fill the jar with water, leaving about 1 inch of space at the top

- Cover the jar with a cloth and secure with a rubber band

- Let the jar sit at room temperature, away from direct sunlight, for 5-7 days, until it tastes tangy and the color is deep red

- Strain out the beets and transfer the liquid to the refrigerator

N.V.: Calories: 40, Fat: 0g, Carbs: 9g, Protein: 2g, Sugar: 7g

HOMEMADE KIMCHI

P.T.: 48 hr | C.T.: 0 min

M. of C.: Fermenting | Serves: 8

Ingr.: 1 medium Napa cabbage, chopped

- 1/4 cup sea salt

- Water to cover

- 2 tablespoons grated ginger

- 4 cloves garlic, minced

- 2 teaspoons sugar

- 3 tablespoons fish sauce

- 1 tablespoon soy sauce

- 1/2 cup Korean red pepper flakes (gochugaru)

- 1 daikon radish, julienned

- 4 green onions, chopped

Proc.: In a large bowl, massage salt into the chopped cabbage until it begins to soften

- Cover with water and let sit for 2 hours to brine

- Rinse the cabbage under cold water and drain thoroughly

- In another bowl, mix together ginger, garlic, sugar, fish sauce, soy sauce, and Korean red pepper flakes to form a paste

- Add the cabbage, daikon radish, and green onions to the paste, ensuring they are well coated

- Pack the mixture tightly into a jar, leaving at least 1 inch of space at the top

- Seal the jar and let it sit at room temperature for 2 days, checking daily to press down the vegetables to keep them submerged under the brine

- After 2 days, taste the kimchi and if satisfied, refrigerate.

N.V.: Calories: 35, Fat: 0g, Carbs: 7g, Protein: 2g, Sugar: 4g

CHAPTER 8: SOUP RECIPES

As we turn the pages to Chapter 7, we immerse ourselves in the comforting embrace of soups. This chapter is not just a collection of recipes; it's a sanctuary for the soul and a haven for health. Soups have the unique power to comfort, heal, and bring people together. In the realm of anti-inflammatory eating, they play a pivotal role, offering a delicious way to deliver a concentrated dose of nutrients, hydration, and warmth.

Here, we explore an array of soups that are as varied in flavor as they are in their health benefits. From soothing broth-based concoctions that whisper promises of comfort on a chilly evening to vibrant, creamy vegetable soups that burst with color and nutrition, each recipe is a testament to the versatility and power of simple ingredients combined with care and intention.

Our journey through these pages will take us beyond the basic, introducing protein-enriched options that satisfy and sustain, alongside plant-based creations that celebrate the bounty of the garden. We pay homage to traditional recipes, infusing them with a twist of modernity and a focus on ingredients that fight inflammation and bolster our immune system.

Whether you're seeking solace in a bowl of warmth, a quick and nutritious meal, or a way to use up the seasonal produce that graces your kitchen, this chapter promises a recipe to match your needs. Let these soups be your guide to a healthier, more flavorful life, where each spoonful carries the power of nature's best medicine.

8.1 SOOTHING BROTH-BASED SOUPS

GINGER CHICKEN ZOODLE SOUP

P.T.: 10 min | **C.T.:** 20 min

M. of C.: Simmering | **Serves:** 4

Ingr.: 1 lb. chicken breast, thinly sliced

- 6 cups chicken broth

- 1 inch ginger, grated

- 2 garlic cloves, minced

- 2 medium zucchinis, spiralized

- 1 carrot, julienned

- 1 red bell pepper, julienned

- 2 Tbls soy sauce

- 1 tsp sesame oil

- Salt and pepper to taste

- Fresh cilantro for garnish

Proc.: In a large pot, bring chicken broth to a simmer

- Add ginger and garlic, simmering for 5 minutes

- Add chicken slices, cooking until no longer pink

- Stir in spiralized zucchini, carrot, red bell pepper, soy sauce, and sesame oil, cooking for another 5 minutes

- Season with salt and pepper to taste

- Garnish with fresh cilantro before serving

N.V.: Calories: 180, Fat: 3g, Carbs: 10g, Protein: 26g, Sugar: 5g

LEMONGRASS BEEF PHO

P.T.: 15 min | **C.T.:** 2 hr

M. of C.: Simmering | **Serves:** 6

Ingr.: 1 lb. beef bones

- 8 cups water

- 2 stalks lemongrass, smashed

- 1 onion, halved and charred

- 3 cloves garlic, charred

- 1 inch ginger, charred

- 2 star anise

- 1 cinnamon stick

- 2 Tbls fish sauce

- Salt to taste

- ½ lb. sirloin, thinly sliced

- Rice noodles, cooked

- Bean sprouts, basil leaves, lime wedges, and sliced chili for serving

Proc.: In a large pot, simmer beef bones in water with lemongrass, charred onion, garlic, ginger, star anise, and cinnamon for 2 hours to make the broth

- Strain the broth, return to the pot, and season with fish sauce and salt

- Arrange cooked rice noodles in bowls, top with thinly sliced sirloin

- Pour hot broth over the sirloin to cook it

- Serve with bean sprouts, basil, lime wedges, and sliced chili

N.V.: Calories: 220, Fat: 5g, Carbs: 20g, Protein: 25g, Sugar: 3g

SIMPLE MISO VEGETABLE SOUP

P.T.: 5 min | **C.T.:** 15 min

M. of C.: Simmering | **Serves:** 4

Ingr.: 4 cups vegetable broth

- ¼ cup miso paste

- 1 cup tofu, cubed

- 1 cup seaweed, chopped

- ½ cup shiitake mushrooms, sliced

- 2 green onions, sliced

- 1 carrot, julienned

- 1 tsp soy sauce

- 1 tsp sesame oil

Proc.: In a pot, bring vegetable broth to a simmer

- In a small bowl, mix miso paste with a little hot broth until smooth, then add back to the pot

- Add tofu, seaweed, mushrooms, and carrot to the pot, simmering for 10 minutes

- Stir in soy sauce and sesame oil

- Garnish with green onions before serving

N.V.: Calories: 100, Fat: 4g, Carbs: 9g, Protein: 6g, Sugar: 3g

TOMATO BASIL CHICKEN SOUP

P.T.: 10 min | **C.T.:** 30 min

M. of C.: Simmering | **Serves:** 4

Ingr.: 1 lb. chicken breast, cubed

- 2 Tbls olive oil

- 1 onion, diced

- 2 garlic cloves, minced

- 4 cups chicken broth

- 1 can (14 oz.) diced tomatoes

- 1 tsp dried basil

- Salt and pepper to taste

- Fresh basil for garnish

Proc.: Heat olive oil in a large pot over medium heat

- Add onion and garlic, sautéing until translucent

- Add chicken and cook until browned

- Pour in chicken broth and diced tomatoes, bringing to a simmer

- Add dried basil, salt, and pepper

- Simmer for 20 minutes

- Garnish with fresh basil before serving

N.V.: Calories: 190, Fat: 6g, Carbs: 8g, Protein: 27g, Sugar: 4g

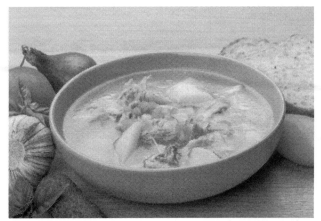

GINGER MISO SEA BASS SOUP

P.T.: 15 min | **C.T.:** 25 min

M. of C.: Simmering | **Serves:** 4

Ingr.: 1 lb. sea bass fillets, cut into pieces

- 4 cups low-sodium vegetable broth

- 2 Tbls miso paste, white

- 1 inch fresh ginger, grated

- 2 garlic cloves, minced

- 1 cup shiitake mushrooms, sliced

- 1 cup bok choy, chopped

- 1 Tbls tamari or low-sodium soy sauce

- 1 tsp sesame oil

- 2 green onions, sliced

- 1 Tbls cilantro, chopped for garnish

- Salt and pepper to taste

Proc.: Dissolve miso paste in a small amount of warm broth to create a smooth mixture

- Heat sesame oil in a pot over medium heat and sauté ginger and garlic until fragrant

- Add vegetable broth, tamari, and miso mixture to the pot and bring to a simmer

- Add sea bass pieces and shiitake mushrooms, simmer gently for 15 min

- Add bok choy and cook for an additional 5 min

- Season with salt and pepper to taste

- Serve garnished with green onions and cilantro

N.V.: Calories: 200, Fat: 6g, Carbs: 10g, Protein: 25g, Sugar: 3g

8.2 CREAMY VEGETABLE SOUPS

CREAMY ROASTED BUTTERNUT SQUASH SOUP

P.T.: 15 min | **C.T.:** 1 hr

M. of C.: Roasting and Blending

Serves: 4

Ingr.: 1 medium butternut squash, halved and seeded

- 2 Tbls olive oil

- Salt and pepper to taste

- 1 onion, chopped

- 3 cloves garlic, minced

- 4 cups vegetable broth

- 1 tsp cinnamon

- ½ tsp nutmeg

- 1 cup coconut milk

- Pumpkin seeds for garnish

Proc.: Preheat oven to 425°F (220°C)

- Brush squash with 1 Tbls olive oil, season with salt and pepper, and place cut side down on a baking sheet

- Roast for 45 minutes until tender

- Sauté onion and garlic in remaining olive oil in a pot until translucent

- Scoop roasted squash into the pot, add vegetable broth, cinnamon, and nutmeg, and bring to a simmer for 15 minutes

- Blend until smooth, stir in coconut milk, and heat through

- Serve garnished with pumpkin seeds

N.V.: Calories: 250, Fat: 14g, Carbs: 33g, Protein: 3g, Sugar: 7g

CARROT GINGER SOUP WITH COCONUT MILK

P.T.: 10 min | **C.T.:** 30 min

M. of C.: Simmering and Blending

Serves: 4

Ingr.: 1 lb. carrots, chopped

- 2 Tbls olive oil

- 1 onion, diced

- 2 Tbls grated ginger

- 4 cups vegetable broth

- 1 can (14 oz) coconut milk

- Salt and pepper to taste

- Fresh cilantro for garnish

Proc.: Heat olive oil in a large pot over medium heat

- Sauté onions until translucent, add carrots and ginger, and cook for 5 minutes

- Pour in vegetable broth, bring to a boil, then simmer until carrots are soft, about 20 minutes

- Blend until smooth, return to the pot, stir in coconut milk, and season with salt and pepper

- Serve garnished with fresh cilantro

N.V.: Calories: 280, Fat: 22g, Carbs: 21g, Protein: 3g, Sugar: 9g

CREAMY MUSHROOM AND WILD RICE SOUP

P.T.: 15 min | **C.T.:** 45 min

M. of C.: Simmering

Serves: 6

Ingr.: 1 cup wild rice, rinsed

- 2 Tbls butter

- 1 onion, chopped

- 2 cups mushrooms, sliced

- 2 cloves garlic, minced

- 1 tsp thyme

- 4 cups vegetable broth

- 1 cup heavy cream

- Salt and pepper to taste

- Fresh parsley for garnish

Proc.: Cook wild rice according to package instructions and set aside

- In a large pot, melt butter and sauté onion, mushrooms, and garlic until tender

- Add thyme and vegetable broth, bring to a simmer, and cook for 20 minutes

- Stir in cooked wild rice and heavy cream, season with salt and pepper, and simmer for another 10 minutes

- Serve garnished with fresh parsley

N.V.: Calories: 300, Fat: 18g, Carbs: 27g, Protein: 7g, Sugar: 4g

CREAMY CAULIFLOWER AND GARLIC SOUP

P.T.: 10 min | **C.T.:** 35 min

M. of C.: Simmering | **Serves:** 4

Ingr.: 1 head of cauliflower, cut into florets

- 2 Tbls olive oil

- 1 onion, diced

- 4 cloves garlic, minced

- 4 cups vegetable broth

- 1 cup coconut milk

- 1 tsp thyme

- Salt and pepper to taste

- Chopped chives for garnish

- Roasted pumpkin seeds for garnish

Proc.: Heat olive oil in a large pot over medium heat

- Add onion and garlic, sautéing until translucent

- Add cauliflower florets, vegetable broth, and thyme

- Bring to a boil, then reduce heat and simmer for 25 minutes or until cauliflower is very tender

- Remove from heat and blend the soup using an immersion blender until smooth

- Stir in coconut milk, and season with salt and pepper to taste

- Serve hot, garnished with chopped chives and roasted pumpkin seeds

N.V.: Calories: 180, Fat: 14g, Carbs: 12g, Protein: 4g, Sugar: 5g

CHICKEN QUINOA SOUP	**BEEF AND LENTIL STEW**

CHICKEN QUINOA SOUP

P.T.: 15 min | **C.T.:** 30 min

M. of C.: Simmering | **Serves:** 4

Ingr.: 1 lb. chicken breast, cubed

- 1 Tbls olive oil

- 1 onion, diced

- 2 carrots, sliced

- 2 stalks celery, sliced

- 4 cups chicken broth

- 1 cup quinoa, rinsed

- 1 tsp turmeric

- 1 tsp garlic powder

- Salt and pepper to taste

- 2 Tbls parsley, chopped

Proc.: Heat olive oil in a large pot over medium heat

- Add chicken and sauté until browned

- Add onion, carrots, and celery, cooking until softened

- Pour in chicken broth and bring to a boil

- Stir in quinoa, turmeric, garlic powder, salt, and pepper

- Reduce heat to a simmer and cook for 20 minutes, or until quinoa is tender

- Garnish with parsley before serving

N.V.: Calories: 320, Fat: 8g, Carbs: 30g, Protein: 30g, Sugar: 3g

BEEF AND LENTIL STEW

P.T.: 20 min | **C.T.:** 1 hr 15 min

M. of C.: Simmering | **Serves:** 6

Ingr.: 1 lb. beef stew meat, cubed

- 2 Tbls olive oil

- 1 onion, chopped

- 3 garlic cloves, minced

- 2 cups beef broth

- 1 cup lentils

- 1 can (14.5 oz) diced tomatoes

- 2 carrots, diced

- 2 tsp thyme

- Salt and pepper to taste

- 2 Tbls fresh parsley, chopped

Proc.: In a large pot, heat olive oil over medium-high heat

- Brown beef on all sides

- Add onion and garlic, cooking until softened

- Pour in beef broth and bring to a boil

- Add lentils, diced tomatoes with juice, carrots, thyme, salt, and pepper

- Cover and simmer for 1 hour, or until beef and lentils are tender

- Garnish with parsley before serving

N.V.: Calories: 380, Fat: 10g, Carbs: 32g, Protein: 38g, Sugar: 4g

SPICY TURKEY CHILI

P.T.: 10 min | **C.T.:** 35 min

M. of C.: Simmering | **Serves:** 6

Ingr.: 1 lb. ground turkey

- 1 Tbls olive oil

- 1 onion, diced

- 2 cloves garlic, minced

- 1 bell pepper, diced

- 1 can (15 oz) kidney beans, drained

- 1 can (15 oz) black beans, drained

- 1 can (28 oz) crushed tomatoes

- 2 Tbls chili powder

- 1 tsp cumin

- 1 tsp smoked paprika

- Salt and pepper to taste

- Fresh cilantro for garnish

Proc.: Heat olive oil in a large pot over medium heat

- Cook turkey until no longer pink

- Add onion, garlic, and bell pepper, sautéing until softened

- Stir in kidney beans, black beans, crushed tomatoes, chili powder, cumin, smoked paprika, salt, and pepper

- Bring to a boil, then reduce heat and simmer for 25 minutes

- Garnish with fresh cilantro before serving

N.V.: Calories: 340, Fat: 8g, Carbs: 38g, Protein: 28g, Sugar: 6g

LENTIL AND TURKEY SAUSAGE SOUP

P.T.: 15 min | **C.T.:** 45 min

M. of C.: Simmering | **Serves:** 6

Ingr.: 1 lb turkey sausage, casings removed

- 2 Tbls olive oil

- 1 onion, diced

- 2 carrots, peeled and diced

- 2 stalks celery, diced

- 3 cloves garlic, minced

- 1 cup green lentils, rinsed

- 6 cups chicken broth

- 1 tsp thyme, dried

- 1 bay leaf

- Salt and pepper to taste

- 2 cups kale, stems removed and leaves chopped

- 1 Tbls apple cider vinegar

Proc.: In a large pot, heat olive oil over medium heat

- Add turkey sausage, breaking it up with a spoon, and cook until browned

- Remove sausage and set aside

- In the same pot, add onion, carrots, celery, and garlic, sautéing until softened

- Add lentils, chicken broth, thyme, bay leaf, salt, and pepper

- Bring to a boil, then reduce heat and simmer for 30 minutes, or until lentils are tender

- Add cooked sausage back to the pot, along with chopped kale, and simmer for an additional 10 minutes

- Stir in apple cider vinegar just before serving

N.V.: Calories: 320, Fat: 10g, Carbs: 35g, Protein: 24g, Sugar: 5g

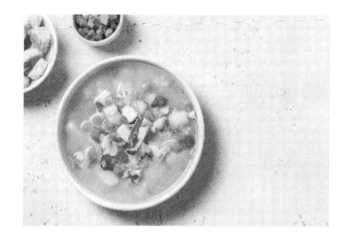

CHAPTER 9: VEGETARIAN RECIPES

In Chapter 8, we journey into the vibrant and wholesome world of vegetarian cuisine, embracing the power of plant-based eating for a life filled with vitality and wellness. This chapter is a testament to the richness and diversity of vegetarian food, proving that a diet free from animal products does not lack in flavor, texture, or nutritional value. Here, we explore an array of recipes that celebrate the bounty of the earth, from the crunch of fresh vegetables to the creaminess of legumes and the hearty satisfaction of grains.

Each recipe is carefully crafted to not only tantalize the taste buds but also to provide a symphony of anti-inflammatory benefits. We delve into the ancient wisdom of spices, the nutritional powerhouse of greens, and the versatile wonders of nuts and seeds. These dishes are designed to nourish the body, soothe the soul, and delight the senses, showcasing how vegetarian meals can be both simple to prepare and profoundly impactful for health.

As we embrace these recipes, we invite you to discover new flavors, textures, and ingredients that perhaps were once foreign but now will become cherished staples in your kitchen. This chapter is more than just a collection of meals; it's a journey towards a more mindful and compassionate way of eating, highlighting the profound connection between our food choices, our well-being, and the health of our planet.

Let this chapter inspire you to explore the endless possibilities that vegetarian cooking offers, empowering you to create meals that are both healing and delicious, and to embrace a lifestyle that celebrates life in its most natural form.

9.1 PLANT-BASED PROTEIN DISHES

CHICKPEA AND SPINACH STUFFED PORTOBELLOS

P.T.: 15 min | **C.T.:** 25 min

M. of C.: Baking | **Serves:** 4

Ingr.: 4 large Portobello mushrooms, stems removed

- 1 can (15 oz) chickpeas, rinsed and drained

- 2 cups spinach, chopped

- 1 garlic clove, minced

- ½ cup red bell pepper, diced

- 1 tsp cumin

- 1 tsp smoked paprika

- Salt and pepper to taste

- ¼ cup tahini

- 2 Tbls lemon juice

- Fresh parsley for garnish

Proc.: Preheat oven to 375°F (190°C)

- Place mushrooms gill-side up on a baking sheet

- In a bowl, mix chickpeas, spinach, garlic, bell pepper, cumin, smoked paprika, salt, and pepper

- Fill each mushroom cap with the mixture

- Mix tahini and lemon juice, drizzle over stuffed mushrooms

- Bake for 25 minutes or until mushrooms are tender

- Garnish with fresh parsley before serving

N.V.: Calories: 220, Fat: 9g, Carbs: 29g, Protein: 9g, Sugar: 6g

LENTIL QUINOA MEATBALLS

P.T.: 20 min | **C.T.:** 30 min

M. of C.: Baking | **Serves:** 4

Ingr.: 1 cup lentils, cooked

- ½ cup quinoa, cooked

- 1 onion, finely chopped

- 2 garlic cloves, minced

- 1 carrot, grated

- 2 Tbls flaxseed meal mixed with 6 Tbls water

- 1 tsp Italian seasoning

- Salt and pepper to taste

- 2 Tbls tomato paste

- 1 cup breadcrumbs

Proc.: Preheat oven to 400°F (200°C)

- In a food processor, combine lentils, quinoa, onion, garlic, carrot, flaxseed mixture, Italian seasoning, salt, pepper, and tomato paste until mixture is well combined but still has some texture

- Stir in breadcrumbs, then form into balls and place on a lined baking sheet

- Bake for 30 minutes, turning halfway through, until golden and firm

- Serve with your favorite pasta sauce

N.V.: Calories: 270, Fat: 3g, Carbs: 49g, Protein: 14g, Sugar: 4g

BLACK BEAN AND SWEET POTATO CHILI

P.T.: 10 min | **C.T.:** 35 min

M. of C.: Simmering | **Serves:** 6

Ingr.: 2 sweet potatoes, peeled and cubed

- 1 can (15 oz) black beans, rinsed and drained

- 1 onion, diced

- 2 garlic cloves, minced

- 1 can (28 oz) diced tomatoes

- 2 Tbls chili powder

- 1 tsp cumin

- 1 cup vegetable broth

- Salt and pepper to taste

- Avocado and cilantro for garnish

Proc.: In a large pot, sauté onion and garlic until translucent

- Add sweet potatoes, black beans, diced tomatoes, chili powder, cumin, vegetable broth, salt, and pepper

- Bring to a boil, then simmer for 30 minutes or until sweet potatoes are tender

- Serve garnished with avocado and cilantro

N.V.: Calories: 200, Fat: 1g, Carbs: 42g, Protein: 8g, Sugar: 9g

TOFU AND BROCCOLI STIR-FRY

P.T.: 15 min | **C.T.:** 10 min

M. of C.: Stir-Frying | **Serves:** 4

Ingr.: 1 lb. firm tofu, pressed and cubed

- 2 Tbls sesame oil

- 1 Tbls ginger, minced

- 2 garlic cloves, minced

- 4 cups broccoli florets

- 1 red bell pepper, sliced

- For the sauce: 3 Tbls soy sauce

- 2 Tbls rice vinegar

- 1 Tbls maple syrup

- 1 tsp cornstarch mixed with 2 tsp water

- Sesame seeds for garnish

Proc.: Heat sesame oil in a large skillet over medium-high heat

- Add tofu cubes and stir-fry until golden on all sides

- Remove tofu and set aside

- In the same skillet, add ginger and garlic, sauté for 1 minute

- Add broccoli and bell pepper, stir-frying until just tender

- Whisk together soy sauce, rice vinegar, maple syrup, and cornstarch mixture to make the sauce

- Return tofu to the skillet, pour in the sauce, and toss to combine and thicken

- Garnish with sesame seeds before serving

N.V.: Calories: 220, Fat: 12g, Carbs: 18g, Protein: 14g, Sugar: 7g

BLACK BEAN AND QUINOA BURGER

P.T.: 20 min | **C.T.:** 10 min

M. of C.: Pan-Frying | **Serves:** 6

Ingr.: 1 cup quinoa, cooked

- 1 can (15 oz.) black beans, drained and rinsed

- 1/2 red onion, finely chopped

- 2 cloves garlic, minced

- 1 carrot, grated

- 1/4 cup cilantro, chopped

- 1 tsp cumin

- 1/2 tsp smoked paprika

- Salt and pepper to taste

- 1 egg (or flax egg for vegan option: 1 Tbls ground flaxseed mixed with 3 Tbls water)

- 2 Tbls olive oil for cooking

Proc.: In a large bowl, mash half of the black beans

- Mix in cooked quinoa, remaining black beans, red onion, garlic, carrot, cilantro, cumin, smoked paprika, salt, and pepper

- Stir in egg or flax egg until well combined

- Form mixture into 6 patties

- Heat olive oil in a pan over medium heat

- Cook patties for 5 minutes on each side or until crispy and golden

N.V.: Calories: 210, Fat: 7g, Carbs: 30g, Protein: 9g, Sugar: 2g

MAPLE GLAZED TEMPEH STIR-FRY

P.T.: 10 min | **C.T.:** 20 min

M. of C.: Stir-Frying | **Serves:** 4

Ingr.: 1 lb. tempeh, cut into 1-inch cubes

- 2 Tbls sesame oil

- 1 red bell pepper, sliced

- 1 cup snap peas

- 1 carrot, julienned

- For the glaze: 3 Tbls maple syrup

- 2 Tbls soy sauce

- 1 Tbls apple cider vinegar

- 1 garlic clove, minced

- 1 tsp grated ginger

- Sesame seeds for garnish

Proc.: Heat sesame oil in a large skillet over medium heat

- Add tempeh cubes and cook until golden brown on all sides

- Remove tempeh and set aside

- In the same skillet, add red bell pepper, snap peas, and carrot, stir-frying until just tender

- Whisk together maple syrup, soy sauce, apple cider vinegar, garlic, and ginger to make the glaze

- Return tempeh to the skillet, pour in the glaze, and toss to coat and heat through

- Garnish with sesame seeds before serving

N.V.: Calories: 320, Fat: 18g, Carbs: 24g, Protein: 20g, Sugar: 12g

BAKED TOFU WITH PEANUT SAUCE

P.T.: 15 min | **C.T.:** 35 min

M. of C.: Baking | **Serves:** 4

Ingr.: 1 lb. firm tofu, pressed and sliced

- For the marinade: 2 Tbls tamari

- 1 Tbls olive oil

- 1 tsp smoked paprika

- For the peanut sauce: ½ cup natural peanut butter

- 2 Tbls lime juice

- 2 Tbls soy sauce

- 1 Tbls maple syrup

- 1 garlic clove, minced

- 1 tsp grated ginger

- Water as needed to thin

- Chopped cilantro and crushed peanuts for garnish

Proc.: Preheat oven to 375°F (190°C)

- Whisk together tamari, olive oil, and smoked paprika

- Marinade tofu slices for at least 10 minutes

- Place tofu on a baking sheet and bake for 35 minutes, flipping halfway through

- For the peanut sauce, combine peanut butter, lime juice, soy sauce, maple syrup, garlic, and ginger in a bowl, adding water to reach desired consistency

- Serve baked tofu drizzled with peanut sauce and garnish with cilantro and crushed peanuts

N.V.: Calories: 290, Fat: 19g, Carbs: 14g, Protein: 21g, Sugar: 6g

SPICY GRILLED TEMPEH SALAD

P.T.: 15 min | **C.T.:** 10 min

M. of C.: Grilling | **Serves:** 4

Ingr.: 1 lb. tempeh, sliced

  - 1 Tbls olive oil

  - 1 tsp chili powder

  - 1 tsp cumin

  - Salt and pepper to taste

  - 4 cups mixed greens

  - 1 avocado, sliced

  - 1 cup cherry tomatoes, halved

  - For the dressing: 3 Tbls balsamic vinegar

  - 1 Tbls Dijon mustard

  - 1 Tbls olive oil

  - 1 tsp maple syrup

  - Salt and pepper to taste

Proc.: Preheat grill to medium-high heat

  - Brush tempeh slices with olive oil and season with chili powder, cumin, salt, and pepper

  - Grill tempeh for about 5 minutes on each side until charred and heated through

  - Toss mixed greens, avocado slices, and cherry tomatoes in a large bowl

- Whisk together balsamic vinegar, Dijon mustard, olive oil, maple syrup, salt, and pepper to make the dressing

  - Arrange grilled tempeh over the salad and drizzle with dressing before serving

N.V.: Calories: 330, Fat: 22g, Carbs: 22g, Protein: 19g, Sugar: 8g

SESAME CRUSTED TOFU WITH SPICY PEANUT SAUCE

P.T.: 15 min | **C.T.:** 20 min

M. of C.: Baking | **Serves:** 4

Ingr.: 1 block (14 oz.) extra-firm tofu, pressed and sliced into 1/2-inch thick slabs

  - 1/4 cup soy sauce

  - 2 Tbls sesame oil

  - 1 Tbls rice vinegar

  - 2 cloves garlic, minced

  - 1 Tbls ginger, grated

  - 1/2 cup sesame seeds

  - For the spicy peanut sauce: 1/4 cup peanut butter

  - 2 Tbls soy sauce

  - 1 Tbls lime juice

  - 1 Tbls honey

  - 1 tsp chili flakes

  - Water to thin

Proc.: Preheat oven to 400°F (200°C)

  - In a bowl, whisk together soy sauce, sesame oil, rice vinegar, garlic, and ginger to create a marinade

  - Dip each tofu slab into the marinade, then coat with sesame seeds

- Place on a baking sheet lined with parchment paper

- Bake for 20 minutes, flipping halfway through, until the tofu is crispy

- For the sauce, whisk together peanut butter, soy sauce, lime juice, honey, and chili flakes, adding water as needed to reach desired consistency

- Serve the tofu hot with spicy peanut sauce on the side

N.V.: Calories: 310, Fat: 22g, Carbs: 14g, Protein: 20g, Sugar: 6g

---

9.3 HEARTY VEGETARIAN CASSEROLES

QUINOA AND BLACK BEAN ENCHILADA CASSEROLE

P.T.: 20 min | **C.T.:** 35 min

M. of C.: Baking | **Serves:** 6

Ingr.: 2 cups quinoa, cooked

- 1 can (15 oz) black beans, rinsed and drained

- 1 can (15 oz) corn, drained

- 2 cups enchilada sauce

- 1 cup Monterey Jack cheese, shredded

- 1 cup cheddar cheese, shredded

- 1 red bell pepper, diced

- 1 green bell pepper, diced

- 1 onion, diced

- 2 cloves garlic, minced

- 1 tsp cumin

- 1 tsp chili powder

- Salt and pepper to taste

- Fresh cilantro for garnish

- Sour cream for serving

Proc.: Preheat oven to 375°F (190°C)

- In a large bowl, combine quinoa, black beans, corn, 1 cup enchilada sauce, half of both cheeses, bell peppers, onion, garlic, cumin, chili powder, salt, and pepper

- Spread half of the remaining enchilada sauce on the bottom of a baking dish

- Add the quinoa mixture and top with the remaining enchilada sauce and cheeses

- Cover with foil and bake for 20 minutes

- Remove foil and bake for an additional 15 minutes until cheese is bubbly

- Garnish with cilantro and serve with sour cream on the side

N.V.: Calories: 350, Fat: 12g, Carbs: 45g, Protein: 18g, Sugar: 5g

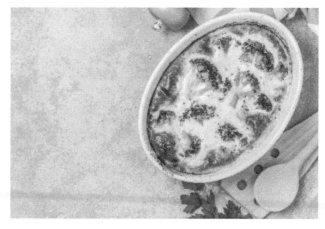

SWEET POTATO AND KALE SHEPHERD'S PIE

P.T.: 25 min | **C.T.:** 30 min

M. of C.: Baking | **Serves:** 6

Ingr.: 4 large sweet potatoes, peeled and cubed

- 1 Tbls olive oil

- 1 onion, chopped

- 2 carrots, diced

- 2 cloves garlic, minced

- 4 cups kale, chopped

- 1 can (15 oz) lentils, rinsed and drained

- 2 Tbls tomato paste

- 1 tsp rosemary, chopped

- 1 tsp thyme, chopped

- Salt and pepper to taste

- ½ cup vegetable broth

- ¼ cup almond milk

- 2 Tbls vegan butter

Proc.: Preheat oven to 375°F (190°C)

- Boil sweet potatoes until tender, then mash with almond milk and vegan butter, season with salt and pepper

- In a skillet, heat olive oil and sauté onion, carrots, and garlic until softened

- Add kale, lentils, tomato paste, rosemary, thyme, salt, pepper, and vegetable broth, simmering until kale is wilted

- Spread lentil mixture in a baking dish, top with mashed sweet potatoes

- Bake for 30 minutes until the top is golden

- Let stand for 5 minutes before serving

N.V.: Calories: 290, Fat: 5g, Carbs: 52g, Protein: 10g, Sugar: 11g

MUSHROOM AND SPINACH LASAGNA

P.T.: 30 min | **C.T.:** 45 min

M. of C.: Baking | **Serves:** 8

Ingr.: 9 lasagna noodles, cooked

- 2 Tbls olive oil

- 1 lb. mushrooms, sliced

- 3 cups spinach, chopped

- 1 container (15 oz) ricotta cheese

- 1 egg

- 2 cups marinara sauce

- 2 cups mozzarella cheese, shredded

- ½ cup Parmesan cheese, grated

- Salt and pepper to taste

- Nutmeg, a pinch

Proc.: Preheat oven to 375°F (190°C)

- Heat olive oil in a skillet and sauté mushrooms until browned, add spinach until wilted

- In a bowl, mix ricotta with egg, salt, pepper, and a pinch of nutmeg

- Spread a layer of marinara sauce in the bottom of a baking dish, layer with noodles, ricotta mixture, mushrooms and spinach, and mozzarella

- Repeat layers, finishing with a layer of noodles, sauce, and sprinkle with Parmesan and remaining mozzarella

- Cover with foil and bake for 30 minutes, remove foil and bake for another 15 minutes until cheese is golden

- Let cool for 10 minutes before serving

N.V.: Calories: 380, Fat: 18g, Carbs: 35g, Protein: 22g, Sugar: 5g

---

SWEET POTATO AND BLACK BEAN CASSEROLE

P.T.: 20 min | **C.T.:** 35 min

M. of C.: Baking | **Serves:** 6

Ingr.: 2 large sweet potatoes, peeled and sliced into 1/4-inch rounds

- 1 can (15 oz.) black beans, rinsed and drained

- 1 red bell pepper, diced

- 1 green bell pepper, diced

- 1 onion, diced

- 2 cloves garlic, minced

- 1 tsp cumin

- 1/2 tsp chili powder

- Salt and pepper to taste

- 1 cup corn kernels, fresh or frozen

- 1 cup shredded cheddar cheese

- 1/4 cup fresh cilantro, chopped for garnish

- 1 avocado, sliced for serving

- 1 lime, cut into wedges for serving

Proc.: Preheat oven to 375°F (190°C)

- In a large bowl, combine sweet potatoes, black beans, red and green bell peppers, onion, garlic, cumin, chili powder, salt, and pepper, tossing to evenly coat

- Layer half of the sweet potato mixture in a greased 9x13 inch baking dish

- Sprinkle half of the corn and half of the cheese over the layer

- Repeat with remaining sweet potato mixture, corn, and cheese

- Cover with foil and bake for 25 minutes

- Remove foil and bake for an additional 10 minutes, or until the sweet potatoes are tender and the cheese is bubbly and golden

- Garnish with cilantro and serve with avocado slices and lime wedges

N.V.: Calories: 280, Fat: 9g, Carbs: 40g, Protein: 12g, Sugar: 7g

CHAPTER 10: SMOOTHIE AND TEA RECIPES

Chapter 9 is a refreshing oasis in our culinary expedition, dedicated to the art of blending and brewing with a focus on smoothies and teas. These aren't just any beverages; they're vibrant elixirs crafted to soothe, rejuvenate, and invigorate your body from the inside out. Here, we explore the delightful synergy between taste and wellness, offering a palette of flavors that are as diverse as they are nourishing.

Smoothies in this chapter are designed to be power-packed meals or snacks, easy to prepare yet filled with the goodness of fruits, vegetables, and superfoods. Each recipe is a testament to the versatility of smoothies, showcasing how a few simple ingredients can transform into a potent concoction for health. From energizing breakfast blends to post-workout refreshers, these smoothies are tailored to support an anti-inflammatory lifestyle, enhancing your body's natural healing processes.

The section on teas delves into the ancient tradition of herbal remedies, highlighting how time-honored brews can offer modern-day wellness solutions. With selections ranging from soothing herbal infusions to robust antioxidant-rich blends, these teas are curated not only for their therapeutic properties but also for their ability to comfort and calm the mind.

As we navigate through Chapter 9, let each sip and slurp serve as a gentle reminder of the powerful connection between what we drink and how we feel. These recipes are more than just beverages; they're a celebration of life's simple pleasures, marrying the joy of drinking with the benefits of living well.

10.1 ANTI-INFLAMMATORY SMOOTHIES

GOLDEN TURMERIC SMOOTHIE

P.T.: 5 min | **C.T.:** 0 min

M. of C.: Blending | **Serves:** 2

Ingr.: 1 C. almond milk

- 1 banana, frozen

- ½ C. mango chunks, frozen

- 1 Tbls chia seeds

- 1 tsp turmeric powder

- ½ tsp ginger, grated

- ¼ tsp cinnamon

- 1 tsp honey, optional

- A pinch of black pepper

Proc.: Combine all ingredients in a blender

- Blend until smooth and creamy

- Pour into glasses and serve immediately

N.V.: Calories: 220, Fat: 4g, Carbs: 44g, Protein: 5g, Sugar: 30g

GREEN GINGER DETOX SMOOTHIE

P.T.: 6 min | **C.T.:** 0 min

M. of C.: Blending | **Serves:** 1

Ingr.: 1 C. spinach, fresh

- ½ C. cucumber, chopped

- 1 green apple, cored and sliced

- ½ banana, frozen

- 1 Tbls fresh ginger, grated

- 1 Tbls parsley, chopped

- 1 tsp lemon juice

- 1 C. water

- 1 tsp spirulina powder

Proc.: Combine spinach, cucumber, apple, banana, ginger, parsley, lemon juice, water, and spirulina in a blender

- Blend until smooth

- Serve immediately for a refreshing detox boost

N.V.: Calories: 180, Fat: 1g, Carbs: 42g, Protein: 4g, Sugar: 25g

SPICY PINEAPPLE AND CUCUMBER SMOOTHIE

P.T.: 8 min | **C.T.:** 0 min

M. of C.: Blending | **Serves:** 2

Ingr.: 1 C. pineapple, chopped

- ½ C. cucumber, chopped

- ½ C. coconut milk

- 1 Tbls lime juice

- 1 tsp chia seeds

- 1/4 tsp cayenne pepper

- 1 Tbls mint leaves, for garnish

- Ice cubes

Proc.: Add pineapple, cucumber, coconut milk, lime juice, chia seeds, and ice cubes to a blender

- Blend until smooth

- Stir in cayenne pepper and blend again briefly

- Serve garnished with mint leaves

N.V.: Calories: 190, Fat: 8g, Carbs: 28g, Protein: 2g, Sugar: 20g

LAVENDER AND CHAMOMILE SOOTHING TEA

P.T.: 5 min | **C.T.:** 10 min

M. of C.: Simmering | **Serves:** 2

Ingr.: 2 Tbls dried lavender flowers

- 2 Tbls dried chamomile flowers

- 4 C. boiling water

- 1 Tbls honey, optional

- Lemon slices, for garnish

Proc.: Place lavender and chamomile in a tea infuser or directly in a pot

- Pour boiling water over the herbs and cover

- Let steep for 10 minutes

- Strain (if herbs were not in an infuser) and serve into cups

- Add honey to taste and garnish with a lemon slice

N.V.: Calories: 35, Fat: 0g, Carbs: 9g, Protein: 0g, Sugar: 8g

GOLDEN GINGER-PINEAPPLE SMOOTHIE

P.T.: 5 min | **C.T.:** 0 min

M. of C.: Blending | **Serves:** 2

Ingr.: 1 C. pineapple chunks, fresh or frozen

- 1 banana, ripe

- 1/2 C. carrots, chopped

- 1 Tbls fresh ginger, grated

- 1 tsp turmeric powder

- 1/4 tsp black pepper

- 1 C. coconut water

- 1 Tbls chia seeds

- 1 tsp honey, optional

Proc.: Combine pineapple, banana, carrots, ginger, turmeric powder, black pepper, coconut water, chia seeds, and honey (if using) in a blender

- Blend on high until smooth and creamy, ensuring the ginger and turmeric are fully incorporated

- If the smoothie is too thick, add a little more coconut water to reach desired consistency

- Serve immediately, garnished with a sprinkle of chia seeds or a pineapple wedge

N.V.: Calories: 180, Fat: 2g, Carbs: 38g, Protein: 3g, Sugar: 25g

10.2 HERBAL TEAS FOR WELLNESS

GINGER TURMERIC IMMUNITY TEA

P.T.: 7 min | **C.T.:** 15 min

M. of C.: Simmering | **Serves:** 2

Ingr.: 1 inch ginger root, thinly sliced

- 1 tsp turmeric powder or 1 inch turmeric root, thinly sliced

- 4 C. water

- Juice of ½ lemon

- 1 Tbls honey, optional

- A pinch of black pepper

Proc.: Bring water to a boil in a saucepan

- Add ginger and turmeric

- Reduce heat and simmer for 15 minutes

- Remove from heat and add lemon juice and black pepper

- Strain into cups and stir in honey to taste

N.V.: Calories: 40, Fat: 0g, Carbs: 10g, Protein: 0g, Sugar: 9g

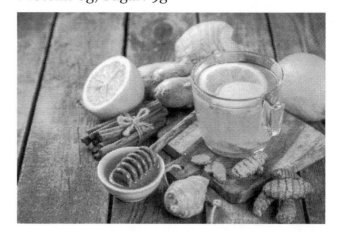

PEPPERMINT AND LICORICE DIGESTIVE TEA

P.T.: 3 min | **C.T.:** 10 min

M. of C.: Steeping | **Serves:** 2

Ingr.: 2 Tbls dried peppermint leaves

- 1 Tbls licorice root, chopped

- 4 C. boiling water

- Lemon wedges, for serving

- 1 tsp honey, optional

Proc.: Combine peppermint leaves and licorice root in a tea pot or large mug

- Pour boiling water over the blend and cover

- Let steep for 10 minutes

- Strain and serve into cups with lemon wedges on the side

- Sweeten with honey if desired

N.V.: Calories: 25, Fat: 0g, Carbs: 6g, Protein: 0g, Sugar: 5g

HOMEMADE ALMOND MILK

P.T.: 8 hr (soaking) | **C.T.:** 10 min

M. of C.: Blending | **Serves:** 4

Ingr.: 1 C. raw almonds, soaked overnight

- 4 C. filtered water

- 2 Tbls maple syrup

- 1 tsp vanilla extract

- A pinch of sea salt

Proc.: Drain and rinse the soaked almonds

- Blend almonds with filtered water until smooth

- Strain the mixture through a nut milk bag or cheesecloth into a large bowl, pressing to extract as much liquid as possible

- Return the milk to the blender, add maple syrup, vanilla extract, and sea salt

- Blend for a few seconds to mix well

- Store in an airtight container in the refrigerator

N.V.: Calories: 60, Fat: 4g, Carbs: 4g, Protein: 2g, Sugar: 2g

SOOTHING LAVENDER CHAMOMILE TEA

P.T.: 5 min | **C.T.:** 10 min

M. of C.: Simmering | **Serves:** 4

Ingr.: 2 Tbls dried chamomile flowers

- 1 Tbls dried lavender flowers

- 4 cups boiling water

- 1 tsp honey, optional

- 1 lemon, sliced for garnish

Proc.: Place chamomile and lavender flowers in a teapot or large infuser

- Pour boiling water over the flowers and let steep for 10 minutes

- Strain the tea into cups, add honey if using, and garnish with a slice of lemon

- Serve hot and enjoy the calming effects

N.V.: Calories: 0 (without honey), Fat: 0g, Carbs: 0g (1g with honey), Protein: 0g, Sugar: 0g (1g with honey)

CINNAMON VANILLA CASHEW LATTE

P.T.: 5 min | **C.T.:** 0 min

M. of C.: Blending | **Serves:** 2

Ingr.: 2 C. homemade cashew milk (see recipe for nut milk preparation)

- 1 Tbls maple syrup

- ½ tsp cinnamon

- 1 tsp vanilla extract

- 1 C. strong brewed coffee, cooled

Proc.: Blend cashew milk, maple syrup, cinnamon, and vanilla extract until smooth

- Pour the mixture into two cups

- Add ½ C. of brewed coffee to each cup

- Stir to combine

N.V.: Calories: 100, Fat: 5g, Carbs: 12g, Protein: 3g, Sugar: 7g

GOLDEN MILK WITH HAZELNUT MILK

P.T.: 10 min | **C.T.:** 5 min

M. of C.: Simmering | **Serves:** 2

Ingr.: 2 C. homemade hazelnut milk

- 1 tsp turmeric powder

- ½ tsp ginger powder

- ¼ tsp cinnamon

- A pinch of black pepper

- 1 Tbls honey, or to taste

Proc.: Warm hazelnut milk in a saucepan over medium heat but do not boil

- Whisk in turmeric, ginger, cinnamon, and black pepper

- Reduce heat and simmer for 5 minutes, stirring occasionally

- Remove from heat, add honey to taste, and stir until dissolved

- Serve warm

N.V.: Calories: 140, Fat: 9g, Carbs: 13g, Protein: 2g, Sugar: 12g

SPICED CASHEW CHAI LATTE

P.T.: 10 min | **C.T.:** 10 min

M. of C.: Simmering | **Serves:** 2

Ingr.: 2 C. cashew milk

- 2 black tea bags

- 1 tsp cinnamon powder

- ½ tsp cardamom powder

- ¼ tsp clove powder

- ¼ tsp nutmeg powder

- 2 Tbls honey

- 1 tsp vanilla extract

Proc.: Bring cashew milk to a gentle simmer in a saucepan over medium heat

- Add tea bags and spices

- Simmer for 10 minutes, stirring occasionally

- Remove from heat and discard tea bags

- Stir in honey and vanilla extract until well combined

- Serve warm, divided into two mugs

N.V.: Calories: 180, Fat: 9g, Carbs: 24g, Protein: 2g, Sugar: 20g

GOLDEN TURMERIC ALMOND LATTE

P.T.: 5 min | **C.T.:** 5 min

M. of C.: Simmering | **Serves:** 2

Ingr.: 2 cups almond milk

- 1 tsp turmeric powder

- ½ tsp cinnamon

- ¼ tsp ginger powder

- 1 Tbls coconut oil

- 1 Tbls honey or maple syrup

- Pinch of black pepper

Proc.: Warm almond milk in a saucepan over medium heat, do not boil

- Whisk in turmeric powder, cinnamon, ginger powder, and coconut oil until fully combined and smooth

- Stir in honey or maple syrup and a pinch of black pepper to enhance turmeric absorption

- Simmer for 5 minutes on low heat, stirring occasionally

- Pour into mugs and serve warm

N.V.: Calories: 150, Fat: 11g, Carbs: 10g, Protein: 1g, Sugar: 8g

CHAPTER 11: DESSERT AND SNACK RECIPES

Embracing an anti-inflammatory lifestyle doesn't mean saying goodbye to desserts and snacks. In fact, it's quite the opposite. Chapter 10 is a sweet revelation that you can indulge in treats that not only satisfy your taste buds but also nourish your body and support your journey towards optimal health. This chapter is dedicated to showing you how to prepare desserts and snacks that are not just healthy but are also irresistibly delicious and easy to make.

From fruit-based desserts that capitalize on the natural sweetness and anti-inflammatory properties of seasonal fruits to snack bars that are perfect for on-the-go nourishment, we've curated recipes that will appeal to everyone in the family. You'll discover guilt-free cookies and muffins that you can enjoy without a second thought, alongside innovative snacks that will make your taste buds dance with joy.

Each recipe has been thoughtfully developed to ensure it's packed with ingredients that fight inflammation, boost your immune system, and provide a burst of energy and nutrition. We've focused on natural sweeteners, whole grains, nuts, seeds, and an abundance of spices to deliver flavor profiles that are both complex and comforting.

Whether you're looking for a quick snack to stave off afternoon hunger pangs or a sumptuous dessert to conclude your meal, this chapter has got you covered. Let's dive into the delightful world of anti-inflammatory desserts and snacks, where health and indulgence meet to create something truly magical.

11.1 FRUIT-BASED DESSERTS

BAKED CINNAMON APPLE CHIPS

P.T.: 15 min | **C.T.:** 2 hr

M. of C.: Baking | **Serves:** 4

Ingr.: 2 large apples, cored and thinly sliced

- 1 tsp cinnamon powder

- 1 Tbls honey

Proc.: Preheat oven to 200°F (93°C)

- Arrange apple slices in a single layer on a baking sheet lined with parchment paper

- Mix cinnamon powder and honey, then brush over apple slices

- Bake for 2 hours, flipping halfway through, until crisp

- Let cool before serving

N.V.: Calories: 95, Fat: 0.3g, Carbs: 25g, Protein: 0.5g, Sugar: 19g

MANGO COCONUT FREEZE

P.T.: 20 min | **C.T.:** 4 hr

M. of C.: Freezing | **Serves:** 6

Ingr.: 2 C. mango, cubed and frozen

- 1 C. coconut milk

- 2 Tbls honey

- ½ tsp lime zest

- Fresh mint leaves, for garnish

Proc.: Blend mango, coconut milk, honey, and lime zest until smooth

- Pour mixture into a loaf pan or silicone molds

- Freeze for at least 4 hours or until firm

- Scoop and serve garnished with mint leaves

N.V.: Calories: 150, Fat: 8g, Carbs: 22g, Protein: 1g, Sugar: 20g

BERRY QUINOA FRUIT SALAD

P.T.: 15 min | **C.T.:** 0 min

M. of C.: Mixing | **Serves:** 4

Ingr.: 1 C. quinoa, cooked and cooled

- 1 C. strawberries, sliced

- 1 C. blueberries

- 1 C. blackberries

- 1 lemon, juice and zest

- 2 Tbls honey

- Fresh mint leaves, for garnish

Proc.: In a large bowl, combine quinoa, berries, lemon juice and zest, and honey

- Gently toss to combine

- Refrigerate until ready to serve, garnished with mint leaves

N.V.: Calories: 210, Fat: 2g, Carbs: 45g, Protein: 6g, Sugar: 15g

CHILLED PAPAYA LIME SOUP

P.T.: 10 min | **C.T.:** 0 min

M. of C.: Blending | **Serves:** 4

Ingr.: 2 C. papaya, cubed

- 1 C. orange juice

- Juice of 2 limes

- 1 Tbls honey

- A pinch of cayenne pepper

- Fresh mint leaves, for garnish

Proc.: Blend papaya, orange juice, lime juice, honey, and cayenne pepper until smooth

- Chill in the refrigerator for at least 1 hour

- Serve cold, garnished with mint leaves

N.V.: Calories: 120, Fat: 0.5g, Carbs: 30g, Protein: 1g, Sugar: 28g

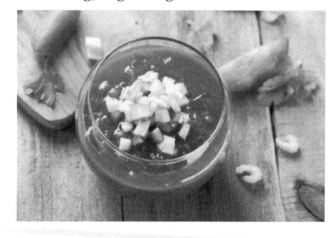

BERRY BLISS FROZEN YOGURT BARK

P.T.: 10 min | **C.T.:** 2 hr (Freezing Time)

M. of C.: Freezing | **Serves:** 8

Ingr.: 2 cups plain Greek yogurt

- 3 Tbls honey

- 1 tsp vanilla extract

- ½ cup strawberries, sliced

- ½ cup blueberries

- ¼ cup raspberries

- 2 Tbls dark chocolate chips

- 1 Tbls shredded coconut

Proc.: In a bowl, mix together Greek yogurt, honey, and vanilla extract until well combined

- Spread the yogurt mixture on a baking sheet lined with parchment paper, creating a layer about ½ inch thick

- Evenly distribute the strawberries, blueberries, raspberries, dark chocolate chips, and shredded coconut over the yogurt layer

- Freeze for at least 2 hours or until completely firm

- Break or cut into pieces and serve immediately

N.V.: Calories: 120, Fat: 2g, Carbs: 18g, Protein: 6g, Sugar: 15g

11.2 HEALTHY SNACK BARS AND BITES

NO-BAKE TURMERIC GINGER ENERGY BITES

P.T.: 15 min | **C.T.:** 0 min

M. of C.: No Cooking | **Serves:** 12

Ingr.: 1 C. rolled oats

- ½ C. almond butter

- ¼ C. honey

- 1 tsp turmeric powder

- 1 tsp ginger powder

- ½ tsp cinnamon

- ¼ C. flaxseeds

- 2 Tbls chia seeds

- ¼ C. unsweetened shredded coconut

Proc.: Mix rolled oats, almond butter, honey, turmeric, ginger, cinnamon, flaxseeds, and chia seeds until well combined

- Form into 1-inch balls

- Roll each ball in shredded coconut until coated

- Chill in the refrigerator until firm

N.V.: Calories: 180, Fat: 10g, Carbs: 20g, Protein: 5g, Sugar: 8g

PUMPKIN SEED & CRANBERRY BARS

P.T.: 20 min | **C.T.:** 25 min

M. of C.: Baking | **Serves:** 10

Ingr.: 2 C. rolled oats

- 1 C. pumpkin seeds

- ½ C. dried cranberries

- ¼ C. honey

- ¼ C. almond butter

- 1 tsp vanilla extract

- ½ tsp salt

- 2 Tbls pumpkin spice

Proc.: Preheat oven to 350°F (177°C)

- Mix rolled oats, pumpkin seeds, and dried cranberries in a bowl

- In a separate bowl, combine honey, almond butter, vanilla extract, salt, and pumpkin spice

- Mix wet and dry ingredients until well combined

- Press mixture firmly into a lined 8x8 inch baking pan

- Bake for 25 minutes or until edges are golden brown

- Let cool before cutting into bars

N.V.: Calories: 210, Fat: 12g, Carbs: 22g, Protein: 6g, Sugar: 10g

DARK CHOCOLATE MATCHA HEMP BITES

P.T.: 15 min | **C.T.:** 0 min

M. of C.: No Cooking | **Serves:** 15

Ingr.: 1 C. dates, pitted

- ½ C. hemp seeds

- ¼ C. cocoa powder

- 1 Tbls matcha powder

- 1 tsp vanilla extract

- A pinch of sea salt

- ¼ C. dark chocolate chips, melted for drizzling

Proc.: Process dates, hemp seeds, cocoa powder, matcha powder, vanilla extract, and sea salt in a food processor until mixture sticks together

- Form into 1-inch balls

- Drizzle with melted dark chocolate

- Chill in the refrigerator until chocolate sets

N.V.: Calories: 160, Fat: 8g, Carbs: 20g, Protein: 4g, Sugar: 14g

TURMERIC CASHEW ENERGY BITES

P.T.: 15 min | **C.T.:** 0 min

M. of C.: No Cooking | **Serves:** 20

Ingr.: 1 cup cashews

- 1 cup Medjool dates, pitted

- 1/4 cup unsweetened shredded coconut

- 2 Tbls chia seeds

- 2 tsp turmeric powder

- 1 tsp cinnamon

- 1/2 tsp ginger powder

- Pinch of black pepper

- 1 Tbls coconut oil

Proc.: Process cashews in a food processor until crumbly

- Add dates, shredded coconut, chia seeds, turmeric, cinnamon, ginger, black pepper, and coconut oil to the food processor

- Blend until mixture sticks together and forms a dough

- Roll the mixture into small balls, about 1 inch in diameter

- Refrigerate for at least 1 hr before serving to set

N.V.: Calories: 100, Fat: 5g, Carbs: 12g, Protein: 2g, Sugar: 9g

11.3 GUILT-FREE COOKIES AND MUFFINS

ZUCCHINI OATMEAL COOKIES

P.T.: 15 min | **C.T.:** 12 min

M. of C.: Baking | **Serves:** 18

Ingr.: 1 C. rolled oats

- 1 C. whole wheat flour

- 1 tsp baking powder

- ½ tsp cinnamon

- ¼ tsp salt

- ½ C. unsweetened applesauce

- ¼ C. honey

- 1 egg

- 1 tsp vanilla extract

- 1 C. zucchini, grated

- ½ C. walnuts, chopped

Proc.: Preheat oven to 350°F (177°C)

- In a bowl, mix oats, flour, baking powder, cinnamon, and salt

- In another bowl, whisk together applesauce, honey, egg, and vanilla extract

- Combine wet and dry ingredients, then fold in zucchini and walnuts

- Drop by spoonfuls onto a baking sheet lined with parchment paper

- Bake for 12 minutes or until edges are golden

N.V.: Calories: 100, Fat: 3g, Carbs: 16g, Protein: 3g, Sugar: 7g

ALMOND FLOUR BLUEBERRY MUFFINS

P.T.: 20 min | **C.T.:** 25 min

M. of C.: Baking | **Serves:** 12

Ingr.: 2 C. almond flour

- 3 eggs

- ¼ C. honey

- 1 tsp baking soda

- 1 tsp vanilla extract

- ¼ tsp salt

- 1 C. blueberries

- Zest of 1 lemon

Proc.: Preheat oven to 375°F (190°C)

- Whisk together almond flour, baking soda, and salt in a large bowl

- In another bowl, beat eggs, honey, and vanilla extract

- Combine wet and dry ingredients, then gently fold in blueberries and lemon zest

- Distribute batter into a muffin tin lined with paper cups

- Bake for 25 minutes or until a toothpick inserted comes out clean

N.V.: Calories: 180, Fat: 11g, Carbs: 15g, Protein: 6g, Sugar: 9g

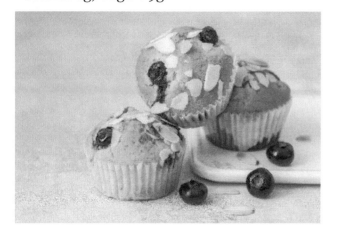

CARROT CAKE QUINOA MUFFINS

P.T.: 25 min | **C.T.:** 20 min

M. of C.: Baking | **Serves:** 12

Ingr.: 1 C. cooked quinoa

- 1 C. whole wheat flour

- ½ C. almond milk

- ¼ C. maple syrup

- 2 eggs

- 1 tsp vanilla extract

- 1 tsp baking powder

- ½ tsp cinnamon

- ¼ tsp nutmeg

- 1 C. grated carrots

- ½ C. raisins

- ¼ C. walnuts, chopped

Proc.: Preheat oven to 350°F (177°C)

- In a large bowl, combine quinoa, flour, baking powder, cinnamon, and nutmeg

- In another bowl, whisk together almond milk, maple syrup, eggs, and vanilla extract

- Mix wet ingredients into dry ingredients until just combined

- Fold in grated carrots, raisins, and walnuts

- Pour into muffin cups and bake for 20 minutes or until an inserted toothpick comes out clean

N.V.: Calories: 150, Fat: 5g, Carbs: 22g, Protein: 4g, Sugar: 10g

ZUCCHINI OAT CHOCOLATE CHIP COOKIES

P.T.: 15 min | **C.T.:** 12 min

M. of C.: Baking | **Serves:** 24

Ingr.: 1 C. grated zucchini, excess water squeezed out

- 1 C. rolled oats

- 1/2 C. almond flour

- 1/4 C. coconut sugar

- 1 tsp vanilla extract

- 1 egg

- 1/2 tsp baking soda

- 1/4 tsp salt

- 1/2 C. dark chocolate chips

- 1/4 C. unsweetened apple sauce

Proc.: Preheat oven to 350°F (175°C)

- In a large bowl, combine zucchini, oats, almond flour, coconut sugar, vanilla extract, egg, baking soda, and salt until well mixed

- Fold in chocolate chips and apple sauce

- Drop spoonfuls of the dough onto a baking sheet lined with parchment paper

- Bake for 12 minutes or until edges are golden

- Let cool on the baking sheet for 5 minutes before transferring to a wire rack to cool completely

N.V.: Calories: 80, Fat: 4g, Carbs: 10g, Protein: 2g, Sugar: 6g

CHAPTER 12: BREAD RECIPES

Bread, in its myriad forms, stands as a cornerstone in diets across the globe, offering comfort, sustenance, and the simple joy of a freshly baked loaf. In **Chapter 11: Bread Recipes**, we're reimagining this staple through the lens of the anti-inflammatory diet, proving that you can indulge in the warmth and satisfaction of bread without straying from your health goals.

Navigating a world where traditional bread often contains ingredients that could exacerbate inflammation, we've crafted recipes that not only exclude these common triggers but also incorporate wholesome, nutrient-dense alternatives. Here, you'll find a collection of breads ranging from gluten-free loaves, rich in flavor and texture, to inventive flatbreads and wraps that incorporate ancient grains and seeds, each offering its unique health benefits.

Our journey through this chapter is not just about substituting or eliminating ingredients; it's about enhancing both the nutritional value and taste of bread. We'll explore how ingredients like almond flour, quinoa, and flaxseeds can transform a simple loaf into a powerful component of an anti-inflammatory diet. Moreover, we introduce fermentation techniques with sourdough recipes, leveraging the gut-health benefits of naturally fermented breads.

Each recipe is designed to be accessible, ensuring that even those new to baking can successfully create their bread at home. With these recipes, we invite you to rediscover the joy of baking bread, turning it into a nourishing act that supports your health, satisfies your palate, and brings warmth to your table.

12.1 GLUTEN-FREE BREADS

ALMOND FLOUR BREAD

P.T.: 15 min | **C.T.:** 40 min

M. of C.: Baking | **Serves:** 0

Ingr.: 3 C. almond flour

- 1 Tbls ground flaxseed

- 1 tsp baking soda

- ¼ tsp salt

- 5 eggs

- 1 Tbls apple cider vinegar

- ¼ C. olive oil

Proc.: Preheat oven to 350°F (177°C)

- In a bowl, mix almond flour, ground flaxseed, baking soda, and salt

- In another bowl, whisk eggs, apple cider vinegar, and olive oil

- Combine wet and dry ingredients until smooth

- Pour into a greased loaf pan

- Bake for 40 minutes or until a toothpick comes out clean

- Let cool before slicing

N.V.: Calories: 280, Fat: 24g, Carbs: 10g, Protein: 12g, Sugar: 2g

COCONUT FLOUR FLATBREAD

P.T.: 10 min | **C.T.:** 15 min

M. of C.: Pan Frying | **Serves:** 0

Ingr.: ½ C. coconut flour

- 2 Tbls psyllium husk powder

- 1 tsp baking powder

- ½ tsp salt

- 1 C. boiling water

- 2 Tbls olive oil

Proc.: Combine coconut flour, psyllium husk powder, baking powder, and salt in a bowl

- Gradually add boiling water and olive oil, mixing until a dough forms

- Divide into 6 balls and flatten each into a disc

- Heat a non-stick pan over medium heat and cook each flatbread for 2-3 minutes on each side until golden brown

N.V.: Calories: 130, Fat: 9g, Carbs: 12g, Protein: 3g, Sugar: 1g

QUINOA AND CHIA SEED BREAD

P.T.: 20 min | **C.T.:** 50 min

M. of C.: Baking | **Serves:** 0

Ingr.: 2 C. cooked quinoa

- ½ C. chia seeds

- ½ C. water

- ½ C. almond flour

- 1 tsp baking powder

- ¼ C. olive oil

- 1 tsp salt

Proc.: Preheat oven to 350°F (177°C)

- Mix chia seeds and water, let sit for 15 minutes until gel-like

- Combine quinoa, chia gel, almond flour, baking powder, olive oil, and salt

- Pour into a lined loaf pan

- Bake for 50 minutes or until firm to the touch and golden

- Let cool before slicing

N.V.: Calories: 200, Fat: 10g, Carbs: 20g, Protein: 6g, Sugar: 0g

BUCKWHEAT AND APPLE CIDER VINEGAR BREAD

P.T.: 15 min | **C.T.:** 60 min

M. of C.: Baking | **Serves:** 0

Ingr.: 2 C. buckwheat flour

- 1 C. almond milk

- 1 Tbls apple cider vinegar

- ½ C. sunflower seeds

- 1 tsp baking soda

- ½ tsp salt

- 2 Tbls maple syrup

Proc.: Preheat oven to 375°F (190°C)

- Mix almond milk and apple cider vinegar, let sit for 5 minutes to curdle

- Combine buckwheat flour, sunflower seeds, baking soda, and salt in a large bowl

- Add curdled milk and maple syrup to dry ingredients, mix until just combined

- Pour into a greased loaf pan

- Bake for 60 minutes or until a skewer comes out clean

- Cool before slicing

N.V.: Calories: 220, Fat: 6g, Carbs: 36g, Protein: 7g, Sugar: 4g

ROSEMARY AND OLIVE OIL GLUTEN-FREE BREAD

P.T.: 15 min | **C.T.:** 40 min

M. of C.: Baking | **Serves:** 0

Ingr.: 2 cups almond flour

- 1 cup tapioca flour

- 1/2 cup ground flaxseed

- 1 tsp baking soda

- 1/2 tsp salt

- 4 eggs

- 1/2 cup olive oil

- 2 Tbls apple cider vinegar

- 1/4 cup water

- 2 Tbls fresh rosemary, finely chopped

- 1 Tbls honey

Proc.: Preheat oven to 350°F (175°C)

- In a large bowl, combine almond flour, tapioca flour, ground flaxseed, baking soda, and salt

- In another bowl, whisk together eggs, olive oil, apple cider vinegar, water, and honey

- Mix wet ingredients into dry ingredients until well combined

- Fold in fresh rosemary

- Pour batter into a greased loaf pan

- Bake for 40 minutes or until a toothpick inserted into the center comes out clean

- Let the bread cool in the pan for 10 minutes before transferring to a wire rack to cool completely

N.V.: Calories: 220, Fat: 14g, Carbs: 18g, Protein: 6g, Sugar: 3g

12.2 HOMEMADE FLATBREADS AND WRAPS

HERBED CHICKPEA FLATBREAD

P.T.: 20 min | **C.T.:** 25 min

M. of C.: Baking | **Serves:** 0

Ingr.: 2 C. chickpea flour (also known as gram flour)

- 2½ C. water

- 1 tsp salt

- ½ tsp black pepper

- 2 Tbls olive oil

- 1 tsp rosemary, finely chopped

- 1 tsp thyme, finely chopped

Proc.: Whisk together chickpea flour, water, salt, and black pepper until smooth and let the batter rest for 15-20 minutes

- Preheat oven to 425°F (220°C)

- Stir olive oil and herbs into the batter

- Pour into a greased baking sheet or cast-iron skillet and spread evenly

- Bake for 25 minutes, or until the edges are crispy and golden

- Cut into pieces and serve warm

N.V.: Calories: 180, Fat: 6g, Carbs: 24g, Protein: 8g, Sugar: 4g

SPELT AND YOGURT WRAPS

P.T.: 15 min | **C.T.:** 5 min

M. of C.: Pan Frying | **Serves:** 0

Ingr.: 2 C. spelt flour

- 1 tsp baking powder

- ½ tsp salt

- 1 C. Greek yogurt

- Water, as needed to form dough

Proc.: Mix spelt flour, baking powder, and salt in a large bowl

- Add Greek yogurt and mix until a dough begins to form, adding water as needed to bring the dough together

- Divide the dough into 8 equal portions and roll each into a thin circle

- Heat a non-stick skillet over medium heat and cook each wrap for about 2-3 minutes on each side or until lightly golden and puffy

N.V.: Calories: 150, Fat: 1g, Carbs: 28g, Protein: 6g, Sugar: 2g

CAULIFLOWER AND ALMOND MEAL TORTILLAS

P.T.: 30 min | **C.T.:** 10 min

M. of C.: Baking | **Serves:** 0

Ingr.: 1 C. cauliflower rice

- 1 C. almond meal

- 2 eggs

- ½ tsp salt

- ½ tsp garlic powder

- ¼ tsp cumin

Proc.: Preheat oven to 375°F (190°C)

- Mix cauliflower rice, almond meal, eggs, salt, garlic powder, and cumin in a bowl until well combined

- Divide the mixture into 6 portions and spread each into a thin circle on a baking sheet lined with parchment paper

- Bake for 10 minutes, flipping halfway through, until edges are slightly crispy

N.V.: Calories: 130, Fat: 9g, Carbs: 8g, Protein: 6g, Sugar: 2g

TURMERIC COCONUT WRAPS

P.T.: 10 min | **C.T.:** 5 min

M. of C.: Pan Frying | **Serves:** 6

Ingr.: 1 cup coconut flour

- 2 Tbls ground turmeric

- 1 tsp sea salt

- 4 eggs

- 1 cup almond milk

- 1/4 cup water

- 2 Tbls melted coconut oil for batter plus more for frying

Proc.: Whisk together coconut flour, turmeric, and sea salt in a large bowl

- In another bowl, beat eggs, then mix in almond milk, water, and 2 Tbls melted coconut oil until well combined

- Gradually pour the wet ingredients into the dry ingredients, whisking continuously until a smooth batter forms

- Heat a non-stick skillet over medium heat and brush with a little coconut oil

- Pour 1/6 of the batter into the skillet, tilting to spread evenly into a thin layer

- Cook for 2-3 minutes on one side, until edges start to lift, then flip and cook for another 1-2 minutes

- Repeat with the remaining batter, adding more coconut oil to the skillet as needed

- Serve warm or allow to cool for later use

N.V.: Calories: 130, Fat: 7g, Carbs: 9g, Protein: 6g, Sugar: 1g

12.3 SAVORY MUFFINS AND SCONES

SPINACH AND FETA MUFFINS

P.T.: 20 min | **C.T.:** 25 min

M. of C.: Baking | **Serves:** 0

Ingr.: 2 C. spelt flour

- 1 Tbls baking powder

- ½ tsp salt

- 1 C. spinach, finely chopped

- ½ C. feta cheese, crumbled

- ¼ C. sun-dried tomatoes, chopped

- 2 eggs

- 1 C. almond milk

- ¼ C. olive oil

Proc.: Preheat oven to 375°F (190°C)

- In a large bowl, mix spelt flour, baking powder, and salt

- Stir in spinach, feta cheese, and sun-dried tomatoes

- In another bowl, whisk together eggs, almond milk, and olive oil

- Combine wet and dry ingredients until just mixed

- Spoon into muffin cups and bake for 25 minutes or until a toothpick comes out clean

N.V.: Calories: 180, Fat: 9g, Carbs: 20g, Protein: 6g, Sugar: 2g

ZUCCHINI CHEDDAR SCONES

P.T.: 15 min | **C.T.:** 22 min

M. of C.: Baking | **Serves:** 0

Ingr.: 2 C. whole wheat flour

- 1 Tbls baking powder

- ½ tsp salt

- ½ tsp garlic powder

- 1 C. zucchini, grated and excess moisture removed

- ¾ C. sharp cheddar cheese, shredded

- ⅓ C. cold butter, cubed

- ¾ C. buttermilk

Proc.: Preheat oven to 400°F (204°C)

- Combine whole wheat flour, baking powder, salt, and garlic powder in a bowl

- Add zucchini and cheddar cheese

- Cut in butter until mixture resembles coarse crumbs

- Gradually add buttermilk, stirring until dough forms

- Turn out onto a floured surface and knead gently

- Cut into 8 wedges and place on a baking sheet

- Bake for 22 minutes or until golden brown

N.V.: Calories: 250, Fat: 14g, Carbs: 24g, Protein: 8g, Sugar: 3g

OLIVE AND ROSEMARY LOAF MUFFINS

P.T.: 20 min | **C.T.:** 30 min

M. of C.: Baking | **Serves:** 0

Ingr.: 3 C. almond flour

- 1 Tbls fresh rosemary, chopped

- 1 tsp baking soda

- ½ tsp salt

- 3 eggs

- 1 Tbls apple cider vinegar

- ½ C. black olives, pitted and chopped

- 2 Tbls olive oil

Proc.: Preheat oven to 350°F (177°C)

- In a bowl, mix almond flour, rosemary, baking soda, and salt

- In another bowl, whisk together eggs, apple cider vinegar, and olive oil

- Combine the wet and dry ingredients, then fold in the olives

- Spoon the batter into muffin cups and bake for 30 minutes or until an inserted toothpick comes out clean

N.V.: Calories: 230, Fat: 19g, Carbs: 10g, Protein: 9g, Sugar: 2g

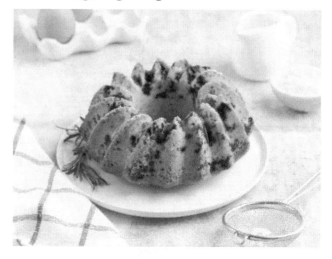

SPINACH AND FETA CHEESE SAVORY MUFFINS

P.T.: 15 min | **C.T.:** 25 min

M. of C.: Baking | **Serves:** 12

Ingr.: 2 C. whole wheat flour

- 1 Tbls baking powder

- 1/2 tsp salt

- 1/4 tsp black pepper

- 1 C. fresh spinach, chopped

- 1/2 C. feta cheese, crumbled

- 1/4 C. sun-dried tomatoes, chopped

- 2 eggs

- 1 C. milk

- 1/4 C. olive oil

Proc.: Preheat oven to 375°F (190°C)

- In a large bowl, whisk together flour, baking powder, salt, and black pepper

- Stir in spinach, feta cheese, and sun-dried tomatoes

- In another bowl, beat eggs, milk, and olive oil together

- Pour the wet ingredients into the dry ingredients and stir until just combined

- Divide the batter evenly among the muffin cups

- Bake for 25 minutes or until the muffins are golden and a toothpick inserted into the center comes out clean

- Let cool in the pan for 5 minutes, then transfer to a wire rack to cool completely

N.V.: Calories: 180, Fat: 9g, Carbs: 20g, Protein: 6g, Sugar: 2g

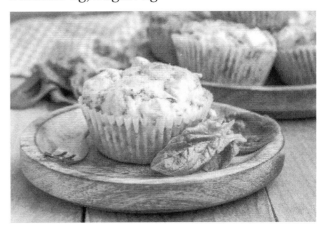

CHAPTER 13: 5 WEEKS TO A HEALTHIER YOU: AN IN-DEPTH MEAL PLAN

Embarking on a journey toward a healthier you can sometimes feel like navigating through a dense forest without a map. The path to wellness is not just about the food we eat; it's about transforming our daily habits, understanding our body's needs, and finding joy in the meals we prepare and savor. In this essential chapter, "5 Weeks to a Healthier You: An In-Depth Meal Plan," we've carefully crafted a comprehensive guide to not just change what's on your plate but to revolutionize your approach to eating and well-being.

Over the next five weeks, we invite you to explore a meticulously designed meal plan that goes beyond mere recipes. It's a journey that introduces you to a symphony of flavors, textures, and nutrients, each playing a crucial role in reducing inflammation and enhancing your overall health. Week by week, you'll discover how simple, delicious meals can be integrated into your lifestyle, making healthy eating not just achievable but utterly delightful.

The first week is about setting the stage, easing you into the anti-inflammatory diet with meals that are both satisfying and simple to prepare. As you progress into the second and third weeks, you'll dive deeper into the heart of anti-inflammatory foods, exploring a variety of ingredients that perhaps were once strangers to your kitchen. Here, the adventure begins, as each meal becomes an opportunity to nourish your body and excite your palate.

By the fourth week, you're ready to embrace the comfort of familiar foods with an anti-inflammatory twist, discovering that healthful eating does not mean sacrificing the flavors you love. Finally, the fifth week is about mastery and celebration. It's about reflecting on the journey, understanding the impacts of your dietary choices, and planning ahead. This is where we equip you with the knowledge and confidence to continue this lifestyle beyond the initial five weeks.

Each week comes with its own set of challenges and triumphs, and we're here to guide you through them. From grocery shopping lists to prep tips and how to handle cravings, this chapter is your compass in the wilderness of healthful eating. Let's begin this transformative journey together, towards a healthier, more vibrant you.

DAY	BREAKFAST	SNACK	LUNCH	SNACK	DINNER
1	GOLDEN TURMERIC MORNING KICK	BAKED CINNAMON APPLE CHIPS	KALE AND QUINOA RAINBOW SALAD	DARK CHOCOLATE MATCHA HEMP BITES	LEMON HERB BAKED SALMON
2	BERRY ANTI-INFLAMMATORY BLAST	MANGO COCONUT FREEZE	BEETROOT AND SPINACH DETOX SALAD	TURMERIC CASHEW ENERGY BITES	SIMPLE GRILLED TILAPIA WITH AVOCADO SALSA
3	GREEN GINGER-PEACH ENERGY	BERRY QUINOA FRUIT SALAD	ASIAN STYLE SLAW WITH GINGER DRESSING	ZUCCHINI OATMEAL COOKIES	OVEN-ROASTED COD WITH CHERRY TOMATOES
4	ANTIOXIDANT ACAI REFRESHER	CHILLED PAPAYA LIME SOUP	WATERMELON AND FETA SALAD WITH MINT	ALMOND FLOUR BLUEBERRY MUFFINS	PESTO-STUFFED TROUT
5	SPIRULINA SUNRISE SMOOTHIE	BERRY BLISS FROZEN YOGURT BARK	KALE AND ROASTED SWEET POTATO SALAD	CARROT CAKE QUINOA MUFFINS	SAFFRON SEAFOOD CHOWDER
6	CINNAMON SPICED QUINOA PORRIDGE	NO-BAKE TURMERIC GINGER ENERGY BITES	CHICKPEA AND TUNA SALAD WITH LEMON VINAIGRETTE	ZUCCHINI OAT CHOCOLATE CHIP COOKIES	TOMATO BASIL SHRIMP STEW

7	ANTI-INFLAMMATORY OATS WITH TURMERIC AND GINGER	PUMPKIN SEED & CRANBERRY BARS	QUINOA AND BLACK BEAN SALAD WITH AVOCADO	ALMOND FLOUR BREAD	LEMONGRASS MUSSELS SOUP

13.2 WEEK 2: DIVING DEEPER INTO ANTI-INFLAMMATORY FOODS

DAY	BREAKFAST	SNACK	LUNCH	SNACK	DINNER
1	BERRY BUCKWHEAT BREAKFAST BOWL	DARK CHOCOLATE MATCHA HEMP BITES	GREEK CHICKEN SALAD WITH HERB DRESSING	SPINACH AND FETA CHEESE SAVORY MUFFINS	MEDITERRANEAN SEAFOOD STEW
2	TURMERIC GINGER OATMEAL	TURMERIC CASHEW ENERGY BITES	CHICKPEA AND QUINOA POWER SALAD	OLIVE AND ROSEMARY LOAF MUFFINS	CITRUS SHRIMP AND AVOCADO SALAD
3	MEDITERRANEAN CHICKPEA SKILLET	ZUCCHINI OATMEAL COOKIES	AVOCADO CILANTRO LIME DRESSING	ZUCCHINI CHEDDAR SCONES	ASIAN CRAB AND CUCUMBER SALAD
4	SWEET POTATO AND KALE HASH	ALMOND FLOUR BLUEBERRY MUFFINS	TAHINI GINGER DRESSING	TURMERIC COCONUT WRAPS	MEDITERRANEAN OCTOPUS SALAD
5	ZUCCHINI AND TOMATO FRITTATA	CARROT CAKE QUINOA MUFFINS	CREAMY DILL AND YOGURT DIP	CAULIFLOWER AND ALMOND MEAL TORTILLAS	SEARED SCALLOP AND GRAPEFRUIT SALAD

6	ANTI-INFLAMMATORY AVOCADO AND EGG BREAKFAST BOWL	ZUCCHINI OAT CHOCOLATE CHIP COOKIES	ROASTED RED PEPPER & WALNUT DIP	SPELT AND YOGURT WRAPS	GINGER-TURMERIC CHICKEN STIR-FRY
7	GOLDEN TURMERIC SMOOTHIE	SPINACH AND FETA MUFFINS	LEMONGRASS BEEF PHO	HERBED CHICKPEA FLATBREAD	LEMONY BASIL TURKEY STIR-FRY

13.3 WEEK 3: EXPLORING GLOBAL ANTI-INFLAMMATORY CUISINES

DAY	BREAKFAST	SNACK	LUNCH	SNACK	DINNER
1	GREEN GINGER DETOX SMOOTHIE	COCONUT FLOUR FLATBREAD	CHICKPEA AND SPINACH STUFFED PORTOBELLOS	SPICY GRILLED TEMPEH SALAD	GINGER CHICKEN ZOODLE SOUP
2	SPICY PINEAPPLE AND CUCUMBER SMOOTHIE	QUINOA AND CHIA SEED BREAD	LENTIL QUINOA MEATBALLS	SESAME CRUSTED TOFU WITH SPICY PEANUT SAUCE	SIMPLE MISO VEGETABLE SOUP
3	LAVENDER AND CHAMOMILE SOOTHING TEA	BUCKWHEAT AND APPLE CIDER VINEGAR BREAD	BLACK BEAN AND SWEET POTATO CHILI	QUINOA AND BLACK BEAN ENCHILADA CASSEROLE	TOMATO BASIL CHICKEN SOUP
4	GOLDEN GINGER-PINEAPPLE SMOOTHIE	ROSEMARY AND OLIVE OIL GLUTEN-FREE BREAD	TOFU AND BROCCOLI STIR-FRY	SWEET POTATO AND KALE SHEPHERD'S PIE	GINGER MISO SEA BASS SOUP

5	GINGER TURMERIC IMMUNITY TEA	CAULIFLOWER AND ALMOND MEAL TORTILLAS	BLACK BEAN AND QUINOA BURGER	MUSHROOM AND SPINACH LASAGNA	CREAMY ROASTED BUTTERNUT SQUASH SOUP
6	PEPPERMINT AND LICORICE DIGESTIVE TEA	TURMERIC COCONUT WRAPS	MAPLE GLAZED TEMPEH STIR-FRY	SWEET POTATO AND BLACK BEAN CASSEROLE	CARROT GINGER SOUP WITH COCONUT MILK
7	CINNAMON VANILLA CASHEW LATTE	SPINACH AND FETA MUFFINS	BAKED TOFU WITH PEANUT SAUCE	SPINACH AND FETA CHEESE SAVORY MUFFINS	CREAMY MUSHROOM AND WILD RICE SOUP

13.4 WEEK 4: COMFORT FOODS WITH AN ANTI-INFLAMMATORY TWIST

DAY	BREAKFAST	SNACK	LUNCH	SNACK	DINNER
1	GOLDEN MILK WITH HAZELNUT MILK	MANGO COCONUT FREEZE	SPICY SZECHUAN CHICKEN STIR-FRY	ZUCCHINI OATMEAL COOKIES	TURMERIC ROASTED CHICKEN WITH VEGETABLES
2	SPICED CASHEW CHAI LATTE	BERRY QUINOA FRUIT SALAD	THAI BASIL CHICKEN STIR-FRY	ALMOND FLOUR BLUEBERRY MUFFINS	BALSAMIC GLAZED TURKEY BREAST

3	GOLDEN TURMERIC ALMOND LATTE	CHILLED PAPAYA LIME SOUP	TURMERIC CHICKEN AND BROCCOLI STIR-FRY	CARROT CAKE QUINOA MUFFINS	LEMON GARLIC HERB ROASTED CHICKEN THIGHS
4	HOMEMADE ALMOND MILK	BERRY BLISS FROZEN YOGURT BARK	CREAMY CHICKEN AND MUSHROOM SOUP	ZUCCHINI OAT CHOCOLATE CHIP COOKIES	HERB-CRUSTED CHICKEN WITH ROASTED VEGETABLES
5	SOOTHING LAVENDER CHAMOMILE TEA	PUMPKIN SEED & CRANBERRY BARS	TURKEY AND SWEET POTATO STEW	ALMOND FLOUR BREAD	BEEF AND LENTIL STEW
6	CINNAMON VANILLA CASHEW LATTE	DARK CHOCOLATE MATCHA HEMP BITES	LEMONGRASS CHICKEN SOUP	COCONUT FLOUR FLATBREAD	SPICY TURKEY CHILI
7	PEPPERMINT AND LICORICE DIGESTIVE TEA	TURMERIC CASHEW ENERGY BITES	LEMON CHICKEN ORZO SOUP	QUINOA AND CHIA SEED BREAD	LENTIL AND TURKEY SAUSAGE SOUP

13.5 WEEK 5: MASTERING MEAL PREP AND PLANNING

DAY	BREAKFAST	SNACK	LUNCH	SNACK	DINNER
1	ANTI-INFLAMMATORY AVOCADO AND EGG BREAKFAST BOWL	BAKED CINNAMON APPLE CHIPS	KALE AND QUINOA RAINBOW SALAD	MANGO COCONUT FREEZE	LEMON HERB BAKED SALMON
2	BERRY BUCKWHEAT BREAKFAST BOWL	DARK CHOCOLATE MATCHA HEMP BITES	ASIAN STYLE SLAW WITH GINGER DRESSING	BERRY QUINOA FRUIT SALAD	GINGER-TURMERIC CHICKEN STIR-FRY
3	SWEET POTATO AND KALE HASH	NO-BAKE TURMERIC GINGER ENERGY BITES	WATERMELON AND FETA SALAD WITH MINT	CHILLED PAPAYA LIME SOUP	OVEN-ROASTED COD WITH CHERRY TOMATOES
4	ZUCCHINI AND TOMATO FRITTATA	PUMPKIN SEED & CRANBERRY BARS	CHICKPEA AND TUNA SALAD WITH LEMON VINAIGRETTE	ALMOND FLOUR BLUEBERRY MUFFINS	LENTIL QUINOA MEATBALLS
5	CINNAMON SPICED QUINOA PORRIDGE	ZUCCHINI OATMEAL COOKIES	GREEK CHICKEN SALAD WITH HERB DRESSING	BERRY BLISS FROZEN YOGURT BARK	BLACK BEAN AND SWEET POTATO CHILI
6	GREEN GINGER-PEACH ENERGY	TURMERIC CASHEW ENERGY BITES	QUINOA AND BLACK BEAN SALAD WITH AVOCADO	ZUCCHINI OAT CHOCOLATE CHIP COOKIES	SIMPLE GRILLED TILAPIA WITH AVOCADO SALSA

7	ANTIOXIDANT ACAI REFRESHER	CARROT CAKE QUINOA MUFFINS	KALE AND ROASTED SWEET POTATO SALAD	SPICED CASHEW CHAI LATTE	CHICKPEA AND SPINACH STUFFED PORTOBELLO

Made in United States
Orlando, FL
14 October 2024

52668856R00063